Have a Baby and Look Better Than Ever

An holistic guide to health and fitness during and after pregnancy

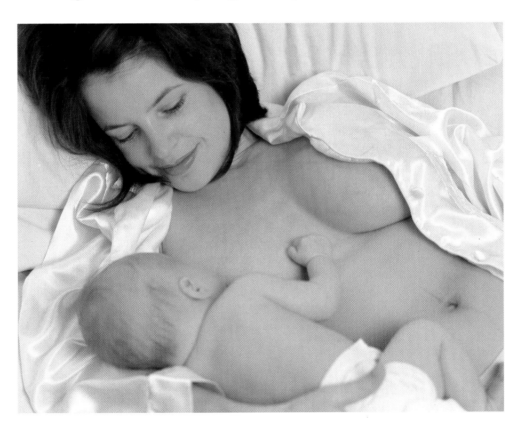

Yinka Thomas and Tonia Buxton

Angel Publications • London

We recommend that before embarking on any of the exercises in this book, the reader seeks approval from her doctor or midwife. Before trying any of the alternative remedies, the reader should seek professional advice from a registered practitioner (see Appendix 2). The book is not intended as a substitute for medical advice.

Published in 2000 by Angel Publications Ltd, London, UK.
Email : angel.publications@virgin.net

Copyright © 2000 Yinka Thomas and Tonia Buxton

Designed by Reece Sutton
Edited by Alison Turnbull

Photography by Patricia Morris using Agfa RSX film
except Chapter 6, Martin Brigdale
Processed by Saints, London

A catalogue record for this book is available from
the British Library

ISBN 0-9536436-0-3

Production by Omnipress, UK
Printed in Spain

For mothers, everywhere.
And Tobi

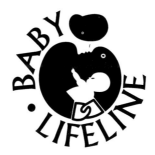

7% of the proceeds of each book sold will be
donated to Baby Lifeline, providing care for
unborn babies,newborn babies and
their mothers throughout the UK.

REG. CHARITY NO: 1006457

Contents

Contents

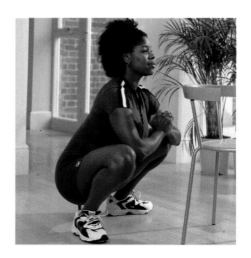

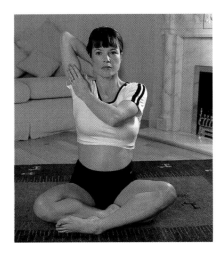
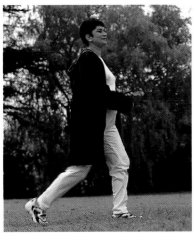
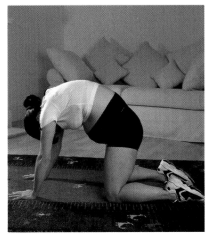

Contributors

Professor Craig Sharp of Brunel University is a physiologist and the UK's leading authority on exercise during pregnancy. He has written widely, and also lectures on the subject.

Dr Mark Stillwell is a GP and father of three who has written a thesis on exercise during pregnancy and its effects. Dr Stillwell has checked the safety of the programme for both mother and child.

Sylvia Baddeley RCM has been a midwife for 26 years and is the author of an exercise in pregnancy book aimed at instructors, midwives, and pregnant mothers. Sylvia is a firm believer in complementary medicine.

The Centre for Nutritional Medicine is run by Drs Beverley and Adam Carey. They use a scientific based understanding of nutrition to improve health, maximise performance, and contribute to disease management and prevention.

Monica McKnight is a health visitor who has visited and advised thousands of new mums.

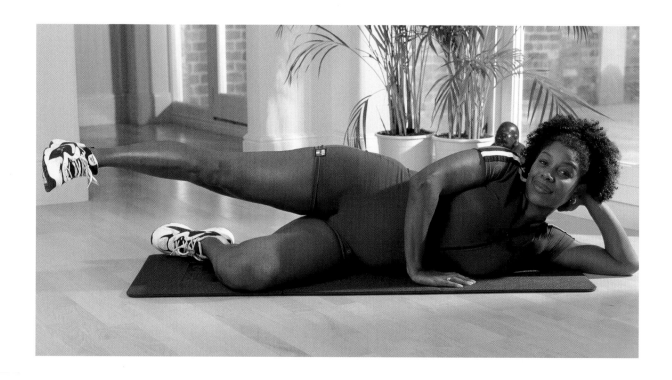

Foreword

I am very pleased to write a foreword for this book on exercise during and after pregnancy. Exercise is one of the most important elements for women caring for themselves before and after the birth of their babies. The others include being well nourished, being in touch with the emotional changes around the time of birth and managing time and sharing care of the baby with friends and family. Meditation and yoga are also extremely useful.

Exercise helps many aspects of women's lives after the birth. It stimulates the endorphin 'love hormones' and makes them feel happy and healthy. It tones and energises the body and protects it from heart disease, diabetes and postnatal osteoporosis. People are surprised at how exercise can reduce the number of hours they need to sleep and increase the amount of energy they have for the birth and for caring for the baby beyond the birth.

I approve of the emphasis in this book on stretching the body, which works very well with yoga postures. I also like the combination of strength training and aerobic conditioning, which makes women look good, reduces the percentage of fat in the body and as the author so eloquently states, provides them with a wonderful tool to enter motherhood feeling attractive and proud of their bodies. I recommend this book because it will not only enhance people's enthusiasm, but it is very practical and the techniques can be used in the comfort on their own home or while walking in the fresh air.

Yehudi Gordon
MB BCh FRCOG FCOG SA

Consultant Obstetrician
The Hospital of St John and St Elizabeth, London
Co-founder of the Active Birth Movement.

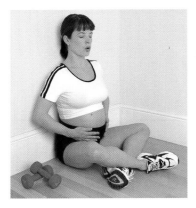 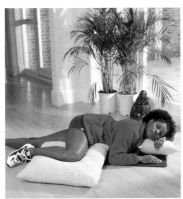 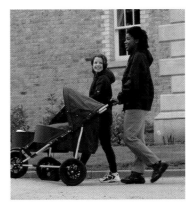

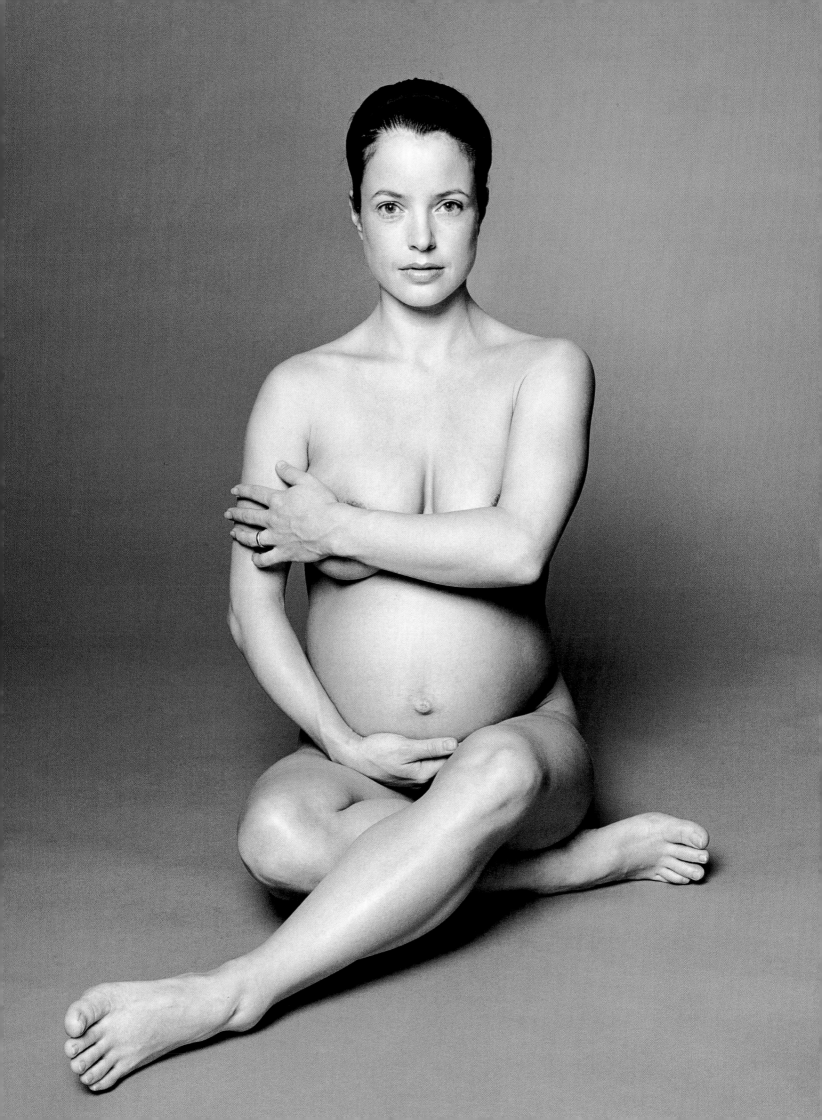

Introduction

This book is a celebration of pregnancy. Myself and Tonia will show you that you can have a baby and look better than ever. Providing a sound scientific basis, we will explore the physiological changes and the wonderful forces of nature that come into play when you are pregnant. We will explain how these changes, when managed by good nutrition and the right type of exercise, can give you a much leaner, toned body after you have had your baby.

But we're also aware that it's all very well saying 'do this type of exercise, eat this and don't eat that, and you'll look great', because that is not the case. True wellbeing is a feeling that comes from the spirit, is realised by the mind, and physically manifests itself in your body and appearance. That is why our approach is holistic

This approach is particularly important at a time when a new mother may be feeling unsure about her body image and ability to cope with motherhood. We put the emphasis back on you after the baby is born, and the aim is that you realise your mental and physical optimum, which is a spiritually enriching experience.

Today, more and more women are taking greater control over their pregnancies, and taking an holistic approach to the whole process. We will explore the psychological changes that you will experience in pregnancy. To feel good about yourself and your appearance, mind, body and spirit have to work in unison, and all three have to be addressed for true wellbeing.

We define wellbeing as:
- a high level of energy
- a desire to maintain physical fitness
- emotional balance
- a sharp mind
- a positive spirit
- and the joy that comes from having all of these qualities.

Pregnancy does not mean the end of a toned, youthful body. It can be the catalyst for a series of body changes that can give you the body you've always wanted. Though it may seem hard to believe, after you have had a baby is the ideal time to re-shape your body, and make it look and feel better than ever. This is because every cell of your body will be motivated to rebuild, tone and repair. There are also psychosocial reasons that make the postpartum period the ideal time to re-train. With such a major life-change, the new mother is open to considering new lifestyle habits. There is a heightened interest in learning and readiness for personal growth.

The book is designed to help you take advantage of this very important time to achieve optimal health, while enhancing your physical appearance and body shape. Though it is most effective when you've just had a baby, it will work for you whether you had your children years ago, or are planning to start a family in the future.

This programme combines what is proven scientifically to be the best method of losing fat, staying slim and looking young. It combines strength training, aerobic conditioning

Introduction

1

through walking, and healthy eating. The basis of the programme involves working with the changes in the pregnant body, rather than against them, to achieve a fitter, well-toned body afterwards. There are no gimmicks, and certainly no diets. We will simply outline the steps to enable you to re-sculpt your body, and reduce fat while adjusting to the emotional changes of the postpartum period.

The benefits to pregnancy and childbirth of physical fitness arising from regular exercise have been known for thousands of years. In Exodus 1.19 two Hebrew midwives explain to the Pharaoh why they cannot carry out his order to kill newborn boys, claiming that Hebrew women are not as the Egyptian women, for they are lively, and are delivered before the midwives come unto them. The Hebrew women were slaves, worked hard and were physically fit, so they had shorter labours than their sedentary mistresses.

Today, women have many pressures: to be good wives, good mothers, home-makers, and have rewarding careers. The last thing we want to do is add to that pressure and say that you must look great after you have had a baby. Pregnancy is the greatest physiological upheaval that the human body has to deal with. What we're saying is that because of the way our bodies work, it is within all of us to work with nature while we are in our most natural state, and to look and feel good after childbirth.

I found I was much leaner after my pregnancy fat had gone, my body was better toned than before (apart from my tummy which I'll write about in Chapter 7). This was as a result of lots and lots of walking. Some days I would walk for over two hours. I'd just wrap the baby up (this was in the middle of winter), and she'd sleep peacefully in the fresh winter air. It was only afterwards, when I first started researching this book, that I discovered the fat burning qualities of walking beats almost all other forms of aerobic exercise. I had literally walked all the baby fat off my body, as well as some of the excess fat that was there before pregnancy and shouldn't have been.

With Tonia the change was more dramatic (see Tonia's story). Tonia had yo-yo dieted for years, tried every diet on the market, even liposuction in a bid to stay slim. After the birth of her first child, she had a brand new body. It was well-toned, strong and firm after strength-training, walking, and healthy eating.

Tonia's story

At the age of 16 I had the type of figure most people would die for, but owing to media conditioning I wanted to be a waif. I felt my bottom and thighs were too big (they weren't). I cleverly decided not to eat for a week, bar a few carrot sticks, lots of black coffee and cigarettes. Here my problems began, putting me firmly in the eating disorder category for the next 12 years of my life.

I lost quite a bit of weight during my starvation week, but as soon as I started eating again, I put it all back on and more, mainly on the my hips and thighs where I least wanted it.

Again I went on a calorie restrictive diet, lost weight (mainly muscle, lowering my metabolism even more), and put it on and more again. I was constantly yo-yo dieting, getting fatter and fatter. It got to the point where I was barely eating anything, doing a lot of aerobic exercise and just getting softer and fatter. My body had gone into starvation mode. When I didn't eat, it thought it was going through a famine, so it would eat away at my muscle and hold on to the fat for survival. When I did eat it would turn the smallest amount of food to fat and store it ready for the next famine. I had made my body inefficient.

Naturally I was very depressed and negative about the way I looked. I felt very weak and there were times when I would black out. I was told that I had hypoglycaemia (low blood sugar) brought on by constant yo-yo dieting. This made my body very sensitive to what I ate. It would over-react and pump out too much insulin, which made me feel very tired and low. Insulin also encourages the body to lay down fat. I really was in a horrible mess: I was fat, my hair was falling out, I was very depressed and unhappy. My insecurity and terrible moods were affecting my relationships with other people, especially my husband. It felt as though there was no way out of this downward spiral.

Then I fell pregnant. During the first few weeks of my pregnancy, before I even knew I was pregnant, I read Yinka's feature in an old copy of *Health and Fitness*. It discussed how various sportswomen had dramatically improved their performances after having children. This article inspired me. I was amazed at the power of the pregnant body.

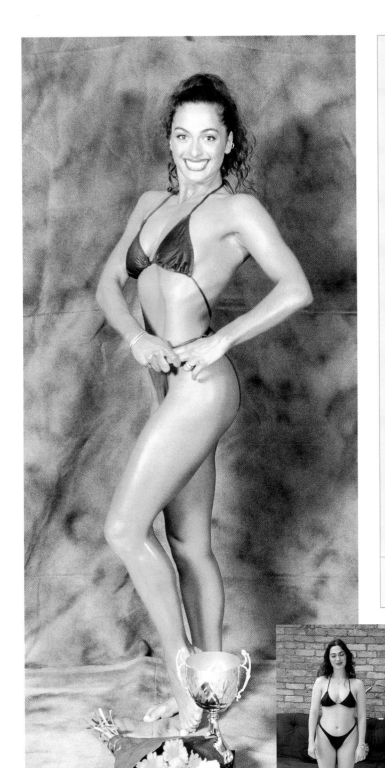

I then discovered I was pregnant and became conscious of the need for a good diet and good exercise, not the manic high intensity aerobic sessions of before. My body seemed to take the cue and heal itself, my blood sugar became constant and I did not have any more energy dips.

I also read about abdominal exercises during pregnancy. The one which struck me most was the simplest, basically having good posture and holding your stomach in. I started doing these exercises regularly. Apart from a little morning sickness and a sensitive nose to horrible smells, I seemed not to get any of the other pregnancy ailments because of healthy diet and exercise. My rings felt much looser on my fingers than they had before I was pregnant.

For me being pregnant was a positive catalyst, both mentally and physically. The thought that I was bringing another human being into the world, who would be dependent solely on me, put my life into perspective. Six months after giving birth to my first child, and at nearly 30 years of age, I had the body I had wanted throughout my late teens and twenties. In fact my waist was smaller than it had ever been before! Just by doing a few exercises, eating well, and being positive.

One year after giving birth I entered and won the Association of Natural Bodybuilders, Miss Athletic of South-East Britain trophy. (The governing body test strictly for steroid users).

The 'before' pictures were taken just months before Tonia became pregnant, and the 'after' pictures were taken while competing at the Association of Natural Bodybuilders competition.

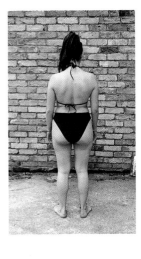

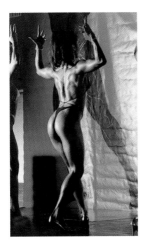

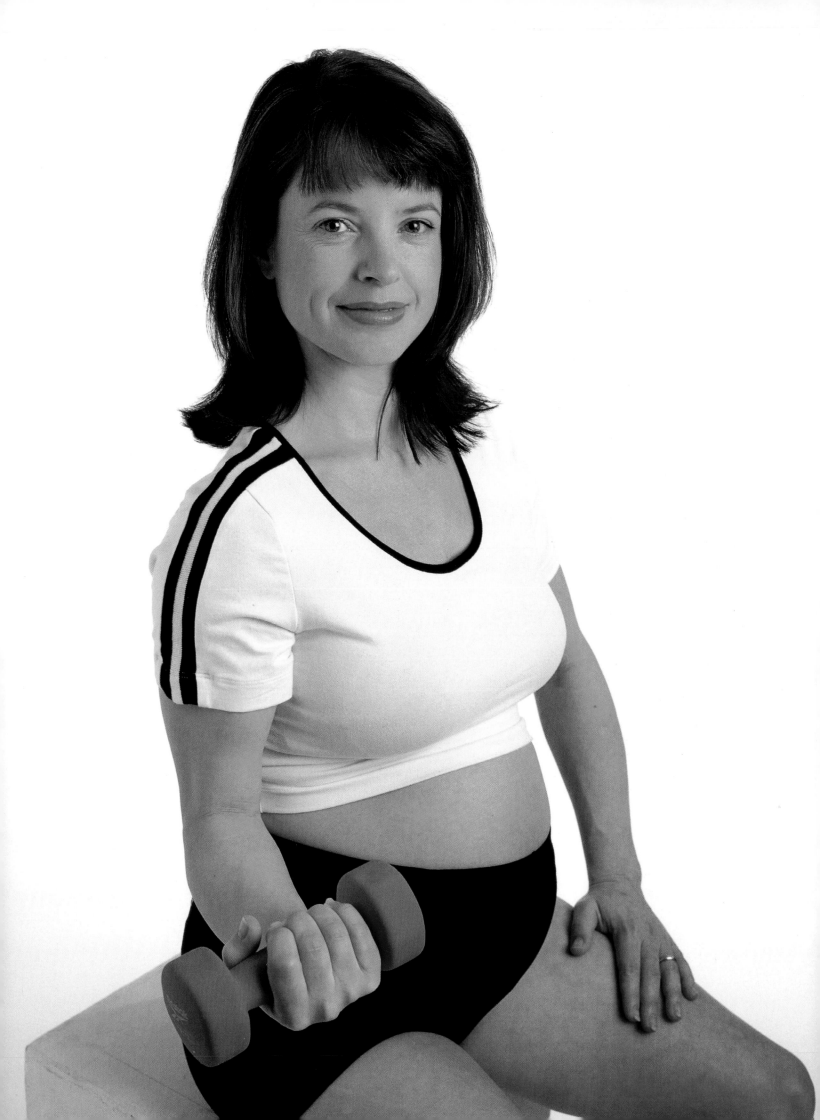

Sporting achievements

Inspiration for the book also came from an article that I wrote for *Health and Fitness* magazine, the same one that Tonia read, about the effects of pregnancy on athletes, particularly long distance endurance runners whose performances seemed to improve dramatically after they had babies.

Ever since Dutch athlete and mother-of-two Fanny Blankers-Koen won four gold medals at the 1948 Olympics, scientists have believed that the best and most natural way for a woman to improve her performance is to have a child.

Some scientists refute this, but the anecdotal evidence speaks for itself. Former women's world marathon record holder Ingrid Kristiansen has two children and won the London Marathon during the period when she was breastfeeding. Norwegian Grete Waitz, the world's best distance runner during the early eighties, achieved many of her famous victories after the birth of her children, and Liz McColgan won the 10,000 metre gold medal at the 1991 world championships nine months after she had given birth to her daughter.

Professor Craig Sharp is a leading sports physiologist at Brunel University and formerly with the British Olympic Medical Centre. Professor Sharp firmly believes in the benefits of childbirth for athletes. He describes pregnancy as progressive resistance training because of the major physiological changes that take place. Professor Sharp says that the positive effects that occur naturally in pregnancy can take years of endurance training to achieve otherwise. Whatever her level of fitness, if a woman trains her body during and after pregnancy, she will become stronger and fitter than before.

Professor Sharp also believes that the work and pain involved in labour leaves you mentally tougher. This is an important quality for a long distance runner who needs to go a little bit faster for that little bit longer. It can also help any woman who has gone through labour to be psychologically stronger.

Having a fit and well-toned body can give a great sense of wellbeing and confidence. During pregnancy, being fit can alleviate leg cramps, back pain, and stress. It can give a sense of control over the many changes taking place in the body, and can give you a positive outlook, not to mention glowing skin.

Benefits of exercise

Everyone – women and men – can benefit from a fitness programme. Box 1 shows some of the general benefits.

Pregnancy places particular demand on a woman's body. Physiologically, pregnancy is the most stressful period of a woman's life, and the demands of a newborn baby can be exhausting. A fitness programme will give you the strength and vitality to make those demands and stresses less exhausting. Box 2 on the next page shows the particular advantages of exercise for pregnant women and new mothers. Many women ask – will exercising make my labour easier? In a study of 250 exercising pregnant women, Hall and Kaufmann[1] found that of those who delivered vaginally, 70% completed third stage labour in less than four hours compared with only 30% of the control group of non-exercising mothers.

The benefits of exercise for everybody	BOX 1

Exercise improves:
- physical shape
- sleep – which becomes deeper and more restful
- bone strength
- endurance
- the immune system – which is better able to fight off infection[2]
- the body's muscle to fat ratio – owing to a small rise in the release of growth hormone[3].

- circulation
- posture
- wellbeing and self-image by reducing tension, anxiety and fatigue
- the body's level of endorphins, a natural chemical that reduces pain and – some say – brightens and lifts the spirits
- youthfulness[4]

Introduction

1

Breathlessness is a common complaint in the later stages of pregnancy. Dr Wolfe and Dr Patricia Ohtake studied 27 previously unfit pregnant women and found that those who spent 20 weeks during their second and third trimesters doing up to 25 minutes of stationary cycling three times a week felt less out of breath than those who remained inactive.

Eighty per cent of the women in this country are sedentary and take no exercise at all[5]. But what we think of as inevitable parts of the ageing process such as:

● lost muscle tone
● stiffness of joints and aches and pains
● decreased strength and flexibility
● middle-age spread
● tiredness
● wrinkles and thinning skin
● decreased stamina and cardiovascular fitness
    are as much a result of being sedentary, as of getting older.

There are many reasons for women not exercising, including lack of time, lack of facilities etc, but one thing that puts many women off is the association of exercise with thinness. Feeling that this socio/cultural ideal is unachievable, many women will not even take up exercise for this reason. This is not our goal. This book is about a healthy lifestyle and true wellbeing that takes very little time and involves no jumping around. With just 15 minutes of strength training three times per week, matched with aerobic conditioning such as walking, you will see some of the many benefits outlined below.

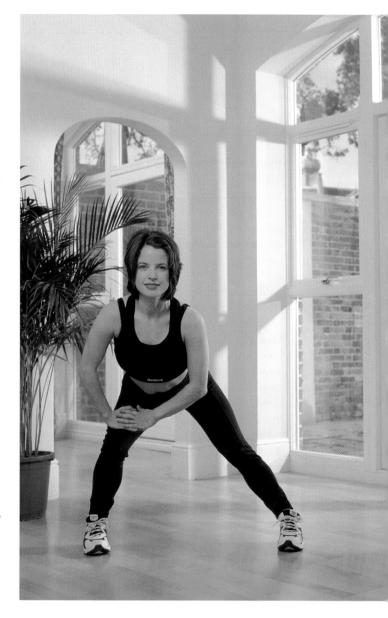

The specific benefits of exercise for pregnant women and new mothers

BOX 2

Exercise:

● helps the body adjust to the growth and recovery stages during and after pregnancy
● increases muscle control and body awareness, creating a positive state of mind, which may help reduce anxiety, fear, and pain
● increases aerobic capacity, which may be helpful for the endurance demands of labour and delivery
● abdominal and back strengthening improves posture and helps prevent postural deviation and its associated discomforts
● helps prevent prolapse of the pelvic organs
● helps reduce pelvic congestions thus preventing cramping and constipation

● helps control weight gain (but should not be used as a means to prevent weight gain)
● may mean a shorter labour and easier delivery (on average two hours less labour time[6])
● improves muscle tone, which helps support the joints and pelvic organs, and leads to a speedier recovery of muscle tone after delivery
● improves balance
● speedier recovery from childbirth
● fewer backaches[7]

Listen to your body

It is very important to listen to your body. It will tell you whether it wants to exercise or do nothing at all. Pearl, one of the mothers photographed in our book, is a dancer. She was very active during her first pregnancy, but when she attempted the same fitness programme during her second pregnancy, despite the strongest will in the world, her body said no. So she did only the minimum of exercise and ate healthily. Don't push yourself. If it doesn't feel good, don't do it.

Giving birth also requires the ability to yield and let go. This means that your body may take over, so you have to work with it rather than try to control it.

Listening to your body and responding to the messages that it gives you is fundamental to wellbeing. When you learn to trust your instincts, you will be surprised how easy it is to do what is right for you. And this is particularly important after childbirth when you will need to recuperate from the pregnancy and delivery.

Rest

When we buy a night cream, the wording on the label will usually say something like 'repairs and nourishes your skin while you are sleeping'. This follows the belief that sleep and relaxation are a time for recuperation, rejuvenation, and repair.

Rest is very important when you are pregnant, and you should try to keep off your feet as much as you can during your final trimester. If you are exercising during this period, it is important that you don't exhaust yourself.

Are there any adverse effects of exercising when pregnant?

Dr James Clapp, who has written widely on exercise during pregnancy, found that children of women who exercised vigorously throughout their pregnancies suffered no harmful effects at all[8]. Researchers who continued to follow this group of babies, found that at five years the children of exercisers had growth in the normal range, though they continued to be somewhat leaner than the children of the non-exercisers. The children of exercisers scored significantly higher than the other children, in tests of intelligence and language skills.

To dispel the myth that exercising mothers produce smaller babies, Dr Maureen Hatch of Columbia University in the United States showed that women who exercise during pregnancy have larger babies who tend to be healthier.

Exercising isn't just good for you it is good for your baby, too.

Getting started

For most people, the difficult part of exercise is starting, and willpower alone is not enough. That is why we are taking an holistic approach. Mind, body and spirit all have to work together to derive maximum benefits. If you start with your mind, the body will follow. Once you've convinced yourself that good nutrition and exercise can make you look younger and feel better and you realise the full potential of just how good you can look physically your body will want to catch up. It will want to get as fit as your mind, and you will start to exercise. When you look good, you feel good, and when you see just how much better you look and feel, you will continue. Because you're looking better, you'll start eating better, and before you know it, without pain or sacrifice, you've changed your life.

It's easy to become sedentary after childbirth. If you're in the house all day, you're burning fewer calories, you may be eating more because you're surrounded by food, breast-feeding makes you hungry, and you may find yourself comfort eating, especially if you've got the 'baby blues'. Just 15 minutes of strength training every other day, and long walks as many times as you can, will make a huge difference.

BACKGROUND INFORMATION ABOUT SOME OF THE ALTERNATIVE REMEDIES WE HAVE RECOMMENDED

Bach Flower remedies

There are 38 Bach Flower remedies, each one dealing with a particular emotional state or aspect of personality. The remedies work on the mental/spiritual level, so they do not interfere with modern medicine. Up to six or seven remedies can be given at one time, depending on need. It is important when diagnosing to take in the person's personality as well as mood in order to treat the whole person. The remedies are preserved in brandy, so it is recommended that they are diluted in water. The Bach Flower remedies can easily be self prescribed but if you have any queries you can call Judy Howard at the Bach Centre and she will give you advice (see Appendix 2, p. 144).

Homeopathy

Homeopathy is an effective and scientific method of healing which assists the natural tendency of the body to heal itself. It recognises that all symptoms of ill health are expressions of disharmony within the whole person and that it is the

Introduction

1

patient that needs treatment not the disease. Hippocrates realised that there were two ways of treating ill health, the way of the opposite and the way of the similar. For example when treating insomnia, the way of the opposite is to treat this by giving a drug to induce artificial sleep. This frequently involves the use of large or regular doses of drugs which can cause side-effects or addiction. The ways of the similar, the homeopathic way, is to give the patient a minute dose of the substance which in large doses causes sleeplessness in a healthy person. Surprisingly this will enable the patient to sleep naturally. Because of the minute dosage, no side-effects or addiction will result.

Homeopathy is subjective: what works for one person may not for another if the emotions are different. So it is very important to go and see a professional homeopath. The remedies in this book are for guidance and can be used safely. When taking a homeopathic cure avoid camphor, coffee, eucalyptus, menthol and peppermint (for example, Vicks or Olbas)

Aromatherapy
The word aromatherapy means 'treatment using scents' and that is exactly what it is. Aromatherapy is a therapeutic and complementary treatment that reaches the very core of our senses through touch and smell, using the scents from aromatic oils to heal and uplift the body and spirit and to make us feel better mentally and physically.

Proper use of the oils helps promote a more balanced lifestyle. There is less likelihood of succumbing to everyday illness and the effects of stress.

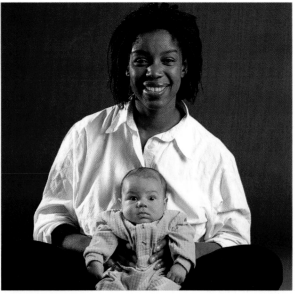

Pearl with Michael

A balanced state of mind promotes vitality and a better ability to cope with potentially difficult events, like coping with a newborn baby. Use of aromatherapy oils can also stimulate the immune system, avoiding that 'run-down' feeling that can cause stress and unhappiness. Remember that you must never use essential oils directly on the skin, and never use them internally.

The mothers featured in the book
The mothers we feature in the book are Pearl Jordan (who we've already mentioned) and Kay Hunter Saber. Pearl is 33 years old, and a dancer, and Michael is her second baby. As with most second pregnancies, she put on a lot more weight than during her first, and also felt unable to exercise as much as she did during her first pregnancy.

Kay, who is 35, is a fitness consultant and Max is her first baby. Kay is an inspiration to us all. Because of her job, Kay is already fitter and a lot more active than most women. However, she shows us how strength training and aerobic conditioning can help you get back into shape after the baby is born. Kay is also a fine testament to how doing the abdominal exercises and proper skin nourishment can get your waist back and tummy flat, which she achieved six weeks after a caesarean section.

We hope that this book will motivate and empower you to experience optimal health, body shape, and appearance. In other words, be the best that you can be. Your self-confidence will be enhanced, and you will be stronger mentally as well as physically, and more effective at accomplishing your goals.

What's in the book
In **Chapter 2** we will explain the scientific studies that have shown strength training to be the best form of exercise to keep you looking young.

Chapter 3 explains the science of fat. How we get fat, and what is the scientifically proven most efficient way of burning excess body fat.

Chapter 4 explores the hormonal, physiological and emotional changes that you will experience during pregnancy, and **Chapter 5** explores the same changes after childbirth. In both chapters we focus on the positive coping strategies for the potential stresses of pregnancy and new motherhood.

In **Chapter 6** we offer a plan for healthy eating but do not include any sort of diet to lose weight. This programme is about shape, not weight.

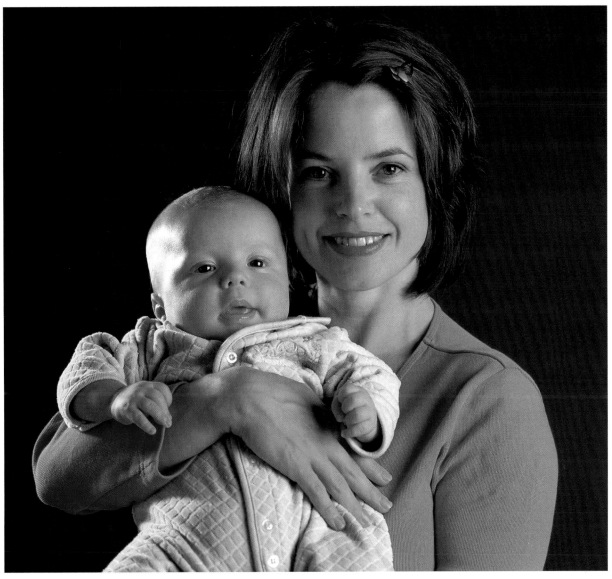

Kay with Max

The waist deserves a chapter in itself **(Chapter 7)**. By concentrating on the waist, even while it is expanding during pregnancy, and by doing certain exercises, the waist can spring back into shape, and often end up smaller than before pregnancy. Chapter 7 also looks at the problem of 'baby belly'. This is the excess skin and fat that remains on the tummy when all the other fat has gone away. It is often a problem with women who have had caesarean sections because the abdominal wall has been cut. It can be difficult and tedious to isolate and exercise the abdominal muscles. We explain how to prevent baby belly, and we look at ways to flatten your tummy if your child is a few years old and you still have it.

Chapters 8 and 9 combine a strength training and an aerobic conditioning programme consisting of walking.

Chapter 10 is all about maintenance, and how to maintain peace of mind, a disciplined body and a healthy spirit. The power of spirit, and a positive frame of mind is just as important to your wellbeing as exercising and good nutrition.

References
1. Hall D., Kaufmann D. (1987) Effects of Aerobic Strength Conditioning on Pregnancy Outcomes. *American Journal of Obstetrics and Gynecology* 157:1199–1203.
2. Sharp N.C.C. (1993) Immunological Aspects of Exercise, Fitness, and Competition Sport. McLeod D.A.D. (Ed) *High Intensity Intermittent Sport E. & F.N. Sport,* p.210.
3. Maughan R., Gleeson M., Greenshaff P. (1997) *Biochemistry of Exercise and Training.* Oxford Medical Publications, p.129.
4. Weeks D., James J. (1998) *Superyoung.* Hodder & Stoughton.
5. *Allied Dunbar National Fitness Survey* (1993) The Sports Council.
6. *American Journal of Public Health* (1998) 88:1528–33.
7. Steinfield S., Quesabery C. *et al.* (1995) Exercise During Pregnancy and Pregnancy Outcome. *Medical Science and Sports Exercise,* 27:634-640.
8. Clapp J.F. (1996) Morphometric and neurodevelopmental outcome at age five years of the offspring of women who continued to exercise regularly throughout pregnancy. *Journal of Paediatrics* 129 (6).

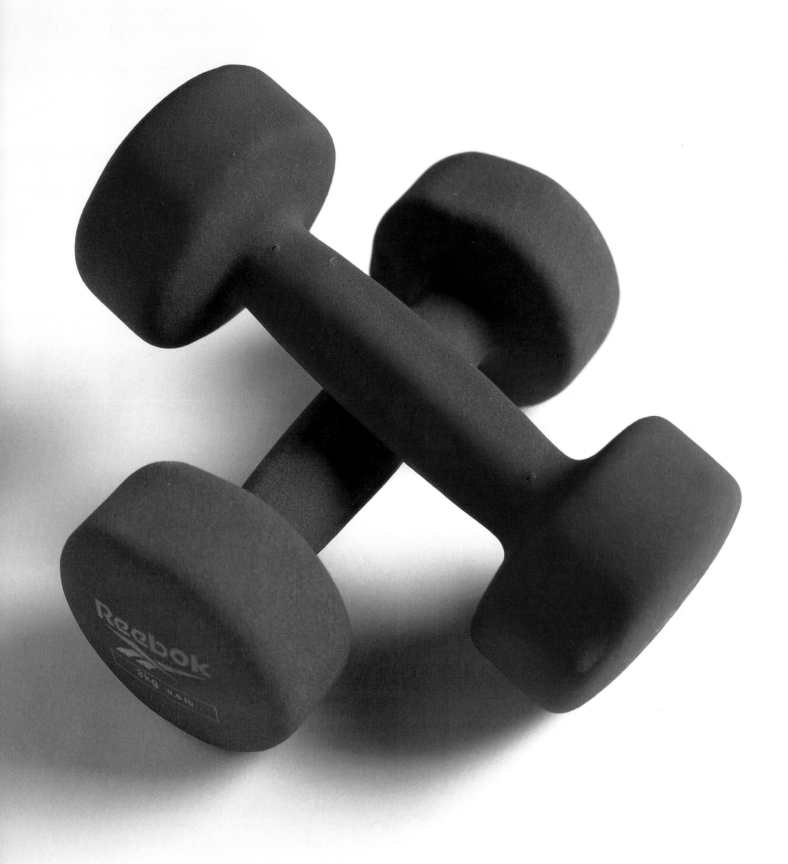

The Science of Strength Training

The programme in this book combines strength training, aerobic conditioning, and optimal nutrition to achieve permanent fat loss and a firm, strong body. Although the fitness programme has been designed specifically for pregnant women and women who have just given birth, all women can use it and benefit.

Exercise and good diet are inextricably linked. Exercising without maintaining a healthy, balanced diet is no more beneficial than good diet and remaining sedentary. The fastest, and most effective way to tone and shape your body is by strength training, and the most efficient and enjoyable way to burn fat is by walking.

Chapter 3 will explain why walking is your best fat burner, this chapter explains why strength training is not only the best way to get a great body, it is also your best anti-ageing weapon.

The benefits of strength training

A humble set of dumbbells is all that you will need to adopt a strength training programme that will keep you slim, keep you young looking, and keep your muscles and bones strong enough to fend off problems like osteoporosis. And there are scientific studies that validate these claims.

This opinion about the benefits of strength training is shown by studies conducted in America, and backed up by medical professionals and organisations including the American College of Sports Medicine, and the American Strength and Conditioning Association.

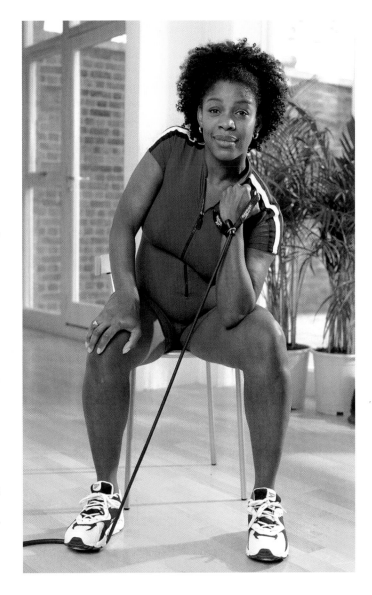

The Science of Strength Training

Strength training increases:
- Muscle strength
- Muscle mass, which makes you more toned
- The body's average calorie-burning rate (metabolism)
- Tendon and ligament strength
- Bone density

Strength training reduces:
- Body fat
- Risk of diabetes
- Risk of osteoporosis
- Blood pressure
- Cholesterol

Strength training improves:
- Balance
- Mood
- Sleep

Well-toned muscles give a body shape and form. Muscle toning firms and tightens. It allows you to change your shape, whether you are developing your arms and shoulders to become less pear-shaped or shaping your legs. Being stronger, and having a well-toned, more disciplined body brings positive psychological effects. You will feel better about yourself. Your self-esteem and self-confidence grow. A strong body brings about a strong mind. Strength training is the key to a better body, and if you combine it with aerobic conditioning, you have the key to a permanently lean body.

How does strength training keep you slim?
Fat accumulates when we eat more calories than we burn. Muscle is the body's most efficient calorie burner. The more muscle we have, the higher our resting metabolic rate – that is, the rate at which our bodies burn calories when we are at rest.

Muscle is metabolically active, and body fat isn't. All muscles vibrate a little 24 hours a day. When these muscles are awoken, they oscillate more, needing to be fed more. This increases your metabolic rate so your body will use food more efficiently.

With the fact that muscle is naturally lost as we get older, it follows that unless we participate in exercise such as strength training, calories don't get burned the way they should, and fat accumulates.

There are several ways to compensate for a metabolism that gets slower as we get older, thus causing the body to lay down fat. We can cut our weekly food intake by 105 calories every year. In 10 years' time, however, we would have to curb our eating by more than 1,000 calories a week. Another option is to add a mile a week – over and above our regular walking workout – every year starting at the age of 30. But by 40, we will have to walk an extra 10 miles per week just to maintain our 21-year-old bodies.

The best option is to add about 60 minutes of strength training per week. And the good thing about this is that you won't have to cumulatively add to your workouts year after year.

A strength training programme will also help to increase cardiovascular fitness. Once you become familiar with the strength training exercises, you will decrease the resting time between sets and increase the weight to keep at your target heart rate.

How does strength training keep you looking young?
As we age, we naturally lose muscle. If we don't challenge our muscles, they will naturally atrophy (waste away) at a rate of about half a pound per year from the age of 20. Even though your weight may stay the same, your body composition will change. You will be the same weight but have more fat and less muscle. This accounts for the frailty associated with those of advanced years.

A lot of this fat accumulates in the tummy region, and has become known as 'middle-age spread'. But a more apt name for it would be 'inactive-muscle induced spread'. Middle-age spread and other signs of ageing are not caused by getting older alone, not exercising our muscles as we get older is as much a reason. And medical advice warns that when a woman's figure plumps to thickness around the middle, her risk of heart disease, diabetes and certain kinds of cancer may also increase. A thickening waist and bulging belly suggest that fat is accumulating around internal organs, and this may underlie the increased health risks.

You can lose weight with aerobics alone, but, very often, and as Tonia found, you'll end up being a 'smaller' version of a flabby person. Significant muscle tone, definition, and strength are rarely achievable from cardiovascular work alone.

You have to use your weights. You need to train your body to be efficient at calorie burning for the other 23$\frac{1}{2}$ hours a day when you're not working out. A person with muscle sitting in front of the television is burning more calories at that moment than a flabby person.

Strength training is simply the most efficient way of increasing lean muscle mass. And while time may conspire against you, you can mount a pretty powerful resistance to its ravages with strength training.

Strength training and osteoporosis

Osteoporosis is a disease which involves a loss of bone density and is associated with ageing. Women are five times more susceptible to osteoporosis than men. The musculoskeletal system slowly becomes weak and brittle, and an accidental fall can mean broken bones or a broken hip.

Research shows that regular strength training and regular weight bearing exercises can increase and maintain bone density thereby reducing a woman's risk of developing osteoporosis, and improving her balance thereby reducing the risk of falls. Regular walking has also been shown to be beneficial.

In addition to this, studies have shown that strength training is safe and effective even for the majority of the senior population. Muscles respond immediately to resistance training and everyone, regardless of age, has the capacity to increase strength.

Strength training and pregnancy

Strength training during pregnancy will give you more stamina and strength during your pregnancy and delivery, and an easier time getting your body back into shape afterwards.

Dr. James Clapp of MetroHealth Medical Centre's Department of Obstetrics and Gynaecology is America's pre-eminent researcher into the benefits of exercise during pregnancy. His research has shown that women who continue to do weight-bearing exercise to at least 50% of their pre-pregnancy capacity can expect to deposit and retain less fat, feel better, control gestational diabetes without insulin, have shorter and less complicated labours, and recover postpartum far quicker than non-exercisers.

There is also the benefit of the mind-body connection. A strong body leads to a strong mind, and can lead to higher self-esteem, and a better sense of control during an unpredictable time of life.

What you will need

You don't need expensive equipment or membership of a health club to strength train. You can start off with just a light set of dumbbells for the during pregnancy exercises

and, as you progress in the postnatal programme, go on to heavier weights.

You will only need about 15-20 minutes, three to four times per week. The key to buying weights is simple: if you like the way something looks and how it feels in your hands, then buy it. Many manufacturers sell sets of dumbbells with 1kg, 2kg and 3kg weights. This may be a useful purchase if you're a beginner. You can start with the lightest weights, and go up a weight as you get stronger.

The basic exercises

The strength training programmes in Chapters 8 and 9 concentrate on muscle toning. You will learn to isolate each muscle and exercise that muscle until it tightens and strengthens. The strong, shapely bodies that we covet are not attainable without good muscle tone, which you get from strength training.

If you're worried that you'll end up as big and muscular as the female bodybuilders you see in muscle magazines, don't. These women train for about 2-4 hours every day, lifting huge amounts of weights, and taking supplements (natural or drugs) to get to the size that they are. Strength training will give you a firmer, toned, more defined body with a good ratio of muscle to fat.

To get started on a good weight-training programme that will give you all of the perceived benefits, you only need seven basic exercises that we include in Chapters 8 and 9.

In those chapters we explain the correct way of doing each exercise. Here we explain what muscles each exercise targets, why it's beneficial, and what it accomplishes.

The basic seven:
● Chest Press
● Back Rows
● Shoulder Press
● Bicep Curl
● Tricep Dips
● Lunges
● Crunches

Chest press

Also known as bench press, this exercise can be done with a chest press machine in the gym, or with dumbbells at home. It targets the muscles of the chest, triceps and front of shoulders. Strong pectoral muscles support your breasts, and are especially important when pregnant because of the extra weight of the breasts. The chest

The Science of Strength Training

press also prevents rounding of the shoulders. When you work your chest you also work your shoulders and triceps.

Back rows

Also known as seated rows, this exercise targets the muscles of the back, specifically the lattissimus dorsi (lats) muscle, and the rhomboids. This can be done on a cable row machine at a gym, or at home using dumbbells for 'bent over rows' or a resistance tube.

Both seated and bent over rows work the lats, rhomboids, and the erector spinae muscles. These muscles when strong, along with the abdominal muscles, support the torso to give good posture. Also by working your lats, you give your back more width, creating a 'v' shape, which in turn makes your waist look smaller.

Shoulder press

Also known as the military press, and seated dumbbell press, it targets the muscles of the shoulders, the deltoids. By working your deltoid muscles, you give your shoulders a square capped off shape, making you look more athletic, and your clothes look better on you. Well developed deltoids make you look broader and your waist look smaller.

Bicep curls

Targets the biceps (front of the upper arms). As well as making you physically strong, good biceps give the arms shape and definition. it also helps if your biceps are strong when you are carrying a growing baby around.

Tricep dips

Targets the triceps (backs of the arms). This muscle at the back of your arm, is one many women feel conscious of. It is the one that flaps when you wave to someone. Strong, firm triceps are a sign of youth, or of training.

Lunges

Lunges and squats target the muscles of the legs (hamstrings) and the bottom (gluteus maximus). This excellent exercise also works the abductor muscles (outer thigh), and adductor muscles (inner thigh). There is nothing better than having a tight firm bottom. This exercise is important if you want to avoid your bottom heading southwards as you get older.

Crunches

Target your abdominal muscles. These and our other abdominal exercises, (especially holding your tummy in), are the tools needed for a tight firm tummy and taut waist. Research has shown that women with thick waists are at

increased risk of heart disease, even if they are of normal weight (from *Journal of the American Medical Association*, December 2 1998). Also strong abdominal muscles, together with a strong back, complete your torso girdle which give good posture. Having a correct posture is essential to achieving good health.

Strength training tips

The general rules for getting started are simple. Start with very light weights, weights that let you complete between 12 and 20 repetitions of the movement. If you can't complete 12, the weight is too heavy. If you can easily do 20, the weight is too light.

Perform between 10 and 15 repetitions (one set) per exercise. Do one set per exercise. Do the routine two to three times a week.

The basic 7 form a great beginner routine that we'll modify as you grow stronger. It will teach your muscles what it's like to move against resistance, and build neural connections between brain and muscle.

Resting time is important. One minute between sets is the optimum since you recover 95% of your strength in that time. Any longer and you will lose the rhythm of your workout, and diminish the benefits.

Progressing

For muscles to get stronger, they need to be continually challenged. Once your body makes the necessary adaptations, after about 6 to 10 weeks of exercise, dramatic muscle change levels off. While you'll still be burning calories, you'll probably stop shedding pounds. For continued muscle growth (and to keep burning fat), alternate lighter weight workouts with heavier ones.

For example, it is good to alternate on a four to six week rotation. For four weeks you do 12 to 15 repetitions in each set and do two sets per exercise, for the light workouts, this also makes your workouts very aerobic and fat burning, as you need less rest time between sets. When you want to do a heavier workout, you are aiming for 8 to10 repetitions for your last set, it would look something like:

- 1kg X 12 repetitions (reasonable weight to warm up the body part with)
- 2kg X 10 repetitions
- 3kg X 8 repetitions (this should be heavy enough so you can just complete your repetitions)

Because your muscle needs recovery time, we recommend that you train each body part once a week (apart from your abdominals, they can be trained every day). Once you decide you wish to make your training a little bit more intense, a training week would look something like this:

Monday:	Abdominals, Back and Biceps
Tuesday:	Abdominals and Aerobics
	(i.e. 20 to 40 minutes brisk walk)
Wednesday:	Abdominals: Chest and Triceps
Thursday:	Abdominals and Aerobics
Friday:	Abdominals, Shoulders, Bottoms and Legs
Saturday:	Aerobics
Sunday:	Rest

Before each strength training session you need to do 10 minutes warm-up aerobics and it is a good idea to end with 10 minutes gentle pace as well. Once you are at this level of training your workouts should be between 45 minutes and 1 hour and 20 minutes.

Once your life is in a better routine and you have been successfully training at home you may wish to progress to a gym. This exercise programme is in itself an excellent introduction to the gym as you already have been using free weights. What the gym would have to offer would be a larger variety of free weights and also weight machines. All gyms will give you an induction programme to show you how to use their equipment. You are no longer a novice of resistance training after doing this programme, but once you start enjoying working out, a gym is a good place to vary your workouts and to socialise. Also many gyms now have good creches for your baby while you train.

Apples or pears

This is a good time to look at your body and decide whether you are happy with that shape. If you are not, there is something you can do about it. There are two basic problem body shapes, the bottom heavy pear or the top heavy apple.

Changing the pear shape

Pear-shaped women hold their fat reserves on their bottoms and legs, and though this is a generally healthier way to hold fat it is not the most aesthetically pleasing, although women of this body shape tend to hold relatively little fat on their abdomen. The classic mistake (and one that Tonia made) is to exercise your bottom half more, lots of cycling and aerobics classes. You only need to look at a professional cyclist to realise this is not the way to go. They have big gluteal muscles and massive thighs but less developed upper bodies. This is because they exercise these muscles so much that they hypertrophy (grow bigger). So what you need to do is the complete opposite.

In order to try and balance our proportions you need to build up your upper body. So your back, and shoulder workouts need to be as heavy as possible. Do not worry about looking like a female body builder, if you are lean and natural it is impossible to look too muscluar. Tonia trained with very heavy weights and did not look 'muscley'. For your bottom half you want to follow the leg routine in the book, with lots of lunges to lift your bottom. Even if you start going to a gym I recommend you stick to these exercises rather than using the machines, you do not need extra resistance, your own body weight is enough to give your bottom and thighs the workout they need, to keep toned but not to build. Training in this way changed Tonia from a pear-shaped body to a well proportioned, toned, lean figure.

Changing the apple shape

Women with this body type hold their body fat on their upper bodies, on their tummy, back and arms. They tend not to have very prominent bottoms and usually have slim legs. High repetitions when working the upper body are needed here. In order to tone your arms you need lots of tricep work, doing two or three sets of 15 to 20 repetitions to keep your arms tight. You will also benefit from doing weighted squats and lunges. Also again looking at the professional cyclist, the stationary bicycle will be good for this body shape, put the gears quite high so it is harder to rotate, as this will tax your legs more, drawing the stores from your upper body into your legs for more shape. If you start to go to the gym, use the leg press and leg curl machines with as much weight as you can.

Stretching

Stretching is important before and after strength training and walking. A few minutes of stretching will make you less likely to injure your muscles. A tight muscle is a vulnerable muscle, and muscles shorten as they fatigue during exercise. Stretching them afterwards gets them back to the pre-workout lengthened position.

Childbirth requires as much the ability to release our muscles as it does to contract them, and to achieve this muscles need to be relaxed and loose, not tight.

Stretching is relaxing and peaceful. It:
● reduces stiffness, muscle tension and soreness
● increases your range of motion
● improves your co-ordination
● improves your posture and balance.
  If you don't stretch because you feel tight you will only get tighter.

The Science of Strength Training

2

Medical check

All of the antenatal and postnatal exercises in this book have been checked and approved by the YMCA Fitness Industry Training – the UK's leading exercise and fitness teacher training organisation, and checked over by Dr Mark Stillwell. But we recommend that you check with your own doctor before starting the exercise programme. Your doctor will know your medical history and, if you have had a baby before, will know how difficult your pregnancy and delivery were. Please also follow the guidelines in Box 3. If you experience any of the danger signs in Box 4, stop exercising immediately and see your doctor as soon as you can.

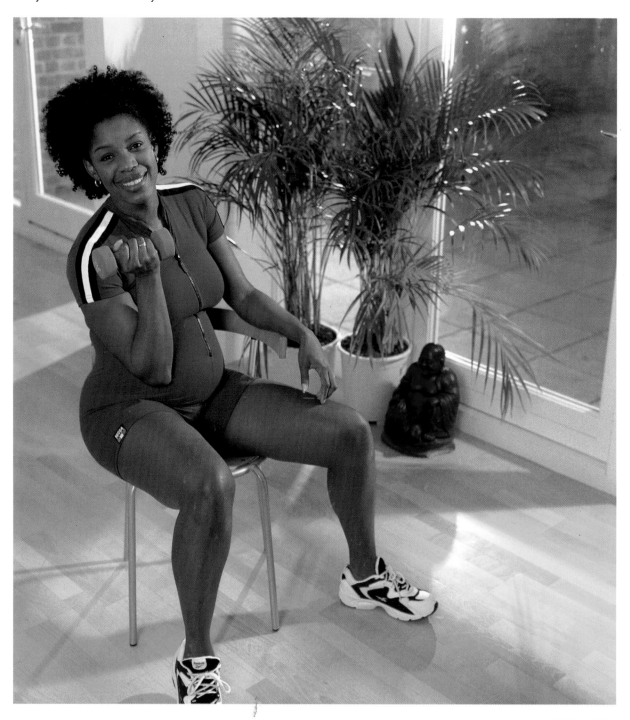

Guidelines for exercising in pregnancy
BOX
3

- You can derive health benefits from as little as 12 minutes, five times a week. Five sessions of 12 minutes, or three sessions of 20 minutes spaced out over a week are better than an hour-long workout only once a week.

- Avoid exercising on your back after the first trimester. Also avoid standing still for long periods. Both can reduce the flow of venous blood to the heart which can make the legs and ankles swell.

- Stop exercising when you become fatigued, and do not exercise to exhaustion.

- Do not hold your breath.

- Do not use heavy resistances after the first trimester. You will make more of the hormone relaxin, which makes body tissue more elastic. Using heavy weights in pregnancy may increase the risk of injury to the joints.

- Most of our exercises are done seated because they are easier to do at any stage of pregnancy

- Avoid exercise in which you could lose your balance, as your centre of gravity moves forward creating instability.

- Avoid any exercise that could cause even mild trauma to the abdomen.

- Avoid invasion games: in contact sports such as netball and hockey an elbow or stick to the abdomen could be dangerous.

- Eat enough food to gain 25-35 pounds over the nine months. We suggest healthy ways of doing this in Chapter 6.

- Avoid overheating, especially in the first trimester. Drink plenty of fluid before and during exercise, wear 'breathable' clothing, do not exercise on hot, humid days, and do not use a hot tub, jacuzzi or sauna.

Danger signs
BOX
4

If you have any of the following, stop exercising immediately. If symptoms persist, contact your doctor or midwife:
- pain of any kind, anywhere
- uterine contractions
- vaginal bleeding or leakage of amniotic fluid
- dizziness or fainting
- shortness of breath
- palpitations or irregular heart beats
- persistent nausea or vomiting
- difficulty walking
- swelling in joints or fingers

Do not exercise while pregnant if:

- you think your baby isn't moving as often as you expect for dates
- you have had pre-term labour in this, or prior pregnancies
- you have persistent vaginal bleeding
- your membranes have ruptured
- you have previously miscarried a baby due to an incompetent cervix
- an ultrasound scan has shown that the fetus is not growing as quickly as it should.

As you work through our postnatal programme, remember these tips:

- *Set realistic goals.* The best way to lose fat and keep it off is to balance the foods you eat with daily physical activity. Losing more than two pounds a week isunhealthy and you are more likely to put the weight straight back on.

- *Magic pills and potions.* There are none, so don't waste your money or your time. If you eat a healthy diet and exercise frequently, excess fat will burn off.
- *Balance diet and exercise.* When it comes to good health

and fat loss, exercise and diet are interrelated. Exercising without maintaining a balanced diet is no more beneficial than dieting while remaining sedentary.

- The beauty of strength training is that you can tailor the programme to aim for the body shape that you want. For example, if you're a classic pear shape, train your upper body – back, shoulders, chest and arms, adding more weight and doing fewer repetitions as you become stronger. To slim the hips and thighs, do more aerobic conditioning such as walking.

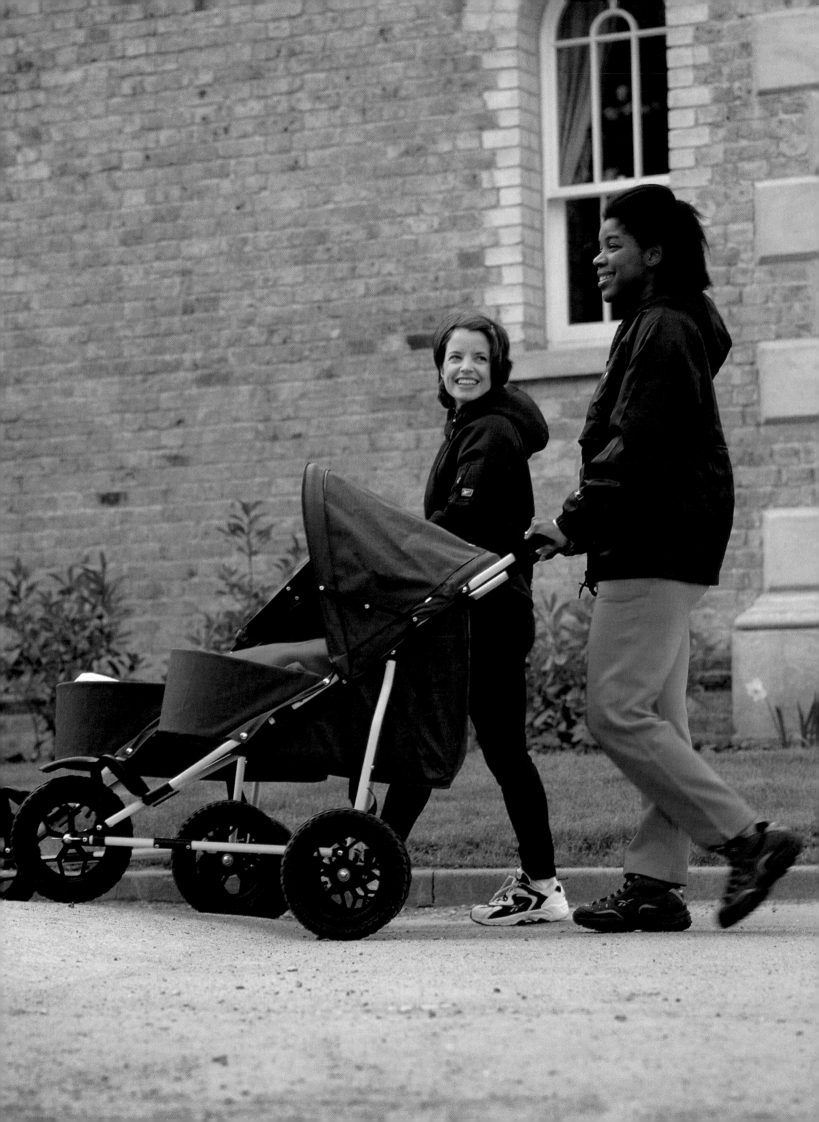

The Science of Fat

I t's natural to gain fat during pregnancy. The weight gained during pregnancy doesn't just round your belly, it puts flesh on your arms, softens your face, gives you curvy hips and bottom and for many a magnificent bosom. Though we firmly believe that you should rejoice in your new, beautiful shape, it is not healthy to carry this extra fat around for ever. We have developed what we believe to be the easiest, safest, and most effective programme to help you lose this fat, and keep it off.

This programme will burn off excess fat whether you had your baby last month, last year, or five years ago. It will even work if you've never had a baby. Here I will explain the 'science' of fat. Why it comes, where it comes from, and how you can get rid of excess fat effectively and permanently, by strength training, good nutrition, and, very importantly, a cardiovascular programme based on walking. As I've said already, our programme is about *fat* loss not *weight* loss. Weight loss achieved by most calorie controlled diets usually results in muscle loss, fluid loss, and bone tissue loss as well as fat loss. This programme is designed for fat loss only.

I won't give a time limit as to how long it will take to lose the fat and have a firm toned body. Setting time limits can be demoralising if you haven't achieved what you want within the given time. As stated in Chapter 1, this is all about listening to your body and working with it. There may

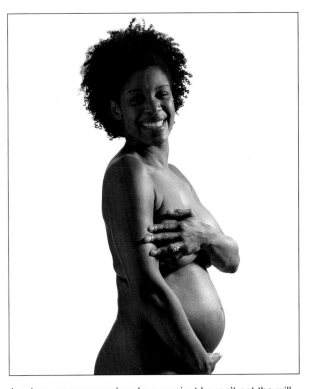

be days, or even weeks when you just haven't got the will to exercise, and may think about nothing but chocolate eclairs. That's all right. What you're aiming to achieve with this programme is not just a temporary plan to rid yourself of excess fat, rather a whole lifestyle change. Eating healthily, toning your muscles by regular strength training, and getting regular cardiovascular exercise. These changes may take a while to become a solid part of your routine, but once you get there and they are as much a part of your routine as going to work and brushing your teeth, you will reap from the positive changes they will bring to your body, mind, and spirit.

The Science of Fat

The Science of Fat

It goes without saying that the less fat we have on our bodies, the more contoured and lean we will look. Just five pounds of excess fat can alter the size of our waists, hips, and thighs so much that clothes are uncomfortably tight.

Fat sits on top of our muscles, so even if we have quite well-toned muscles, no-one will ever know because they can't see them. Fat can latch on to the side of your hips and thighs making you appear wide and pear-shaped, and can produce the dimpled effect commonly known as cellulite.

Fat can be visceral, or subcutaneous. Visceral fat is deep, hard fat that surrounds your internal organs and contributes to a thick waist. Visceral fat has been associated with heart disease and diabetes. Subcutaneous fat is the kind that lays just beneath your skin. Though not as harmful, subcutaneous fat is what makes you look flabby.

We all have a set number of fat cells. Lean individuals have between 20 and 40 billion. Fat cells do not go away. They either shrink or expand as we lose or gain fat. Whatever you eat during the day, which is beyond what you are able to burn, is converted to fat and stored in your fat cells causing them to expand. However, there are several times during the life cycle when the body is receptive to the accumulation of new fat cells:

Infancy

The first time after birth when additional fat cells are produced is during the first year of life. As long as a baby is fed a nutritious diet, they are not likely to gain an unhealthy number of new fat cells.

> **'Fat-Proofing' your Baby**
> ● Breast feeding has many proven benefits, studies have shown that a breast-fed infant is less likely to be an obese child and adult. An American study found that of a group of obese children, 95% had not been breast-fed[1].
>
> ● Breast-fed infants are leaner than formula-fed infants at one year. The formula-fed infants were fatter because energy intake on high carbohydrate formula feed is higher[2]. Breast milk contains human Epidermal Growth Factor (EGF), a potent inhibitor of obesity not present in infant formula and cow's milk.
>
> ● Also to fat-proof your child, expectant mothers should limit carbohydrate and sugar consumption during pregnancy and lactation to prevent excessive insulin levels. And infants should not be fed too high a carbohydrate diet.

Adolescence

The second time when fat cells are susceptible to accumulating and expanding is during adolescence. Many teenagers consume large amounts of sugar and fat from junk food and this is a very vulnerable time for fat weight gain.

Pregnancy

The next crucial period when there is a tendency to synthesise new fat cells is during the third trimester of pregnancy. The first hormonal changes that occur with pregnancy redirect the mother's metabolism to fat storage and fat use, saving the carbohydrates for the developing fetus.

Some fat gain during pregnancy is vital. Eating healthily and taking some exercise will prevent this increase from going above what is necessary. Fat cells may be added at other times during adulthood. One speculation is that 'yo-yo' dieting may cause an increase in fat cell numbers. There have also been reports that liposuction from one area can lead to fat cell gain in other areas[3] (Tonia can testify to this!). This may be because reverting back to normal eating and lifestyle causes fat cells to expand in other areas after certain ones have been removed.

Learning to maintain healthy eating practices and getting some exercise, particularly during the times when fat cells are more likely to be synthesised, may be the best way to avoid gaining fat weight that can be hard to shift later.

The bathroom scales don't tell the whole story

Unfortunately, our civilisation has been brainwashed into believing that weight is the most important factor in terms of health. What really matters, however, is body composition. Weight does not take into account the composition of the body.

Instead of worrying about weight loss, you should be concentrating on fat loss. When you're working towards a goal, it's important to evaluate your progress regularly. The usual way of measuring progress with most calorie controlled diets is to head for the scales. Don't. Weighing yourself daily can be misleading, even damaging. It may encourage you if you are losing weight, but can be dispiriting if you're not, and your confidence will plummet. Weight loss is not a true reflection of the progress you are making in losing body fat. As a barometer for measuring progress, use inches rather than pounds. A reminder that this programme is about shape not weight. When you are pregnant, it is important to monitor weight gain regularly. But after you've had your baby, restrict weighing yourself to just occasionally, after you have seen some progress by simply looking at yourself naked in a full length mirror. If what you see is firm, toned and animated, you're already there. If it's not, focus on:

● getting your body fat percentage down
● getting stronger and fitter
● losing inches
● making progress in your workouts.

If you do this, you will get a truer reflection of your progress. Although it takes up less space, muscle weighs more than fat. If you have always been slim, and take up strength training which results in a strong, well-toned body with a low fat to muscle ratio, you will weigh more than when you had a higher fat to muscle ratio.

Though it sounds paradoxical, you can be skinny and fat. Have you ever wondered why so many catwalk models are only too pleased to bare their boobs, but will never show their bottoms. it's because many of them have the dimply fat on their bottoms and thighs known as cellulite. An unhealthy diet, and inadequate body toning gives them a high fat to muscle ratio.

The best guide to how well you are doing is to use a full length mirror and a tape measure, and measure your body fat. Your level of body fat will tell you what you can already see in your mirror, whether you need to lower it, and where from. Using a tape measure is very useful. As muscle is denser than fat, generally speaking, if your measurements are decreasing, you are losing fat. Good sites for taking measurements are the waist, hips and thighs as these are the typical sites of fat accumulation. You should always place the tape measure in the same place. Use your belly-button for the waist measurement, and fullest part of your buttocks for the hips. Measurements should not be taken more often than once a fortnight. Changes may take some time to appear and taking measurements more often than this may lead to frustration from lack of results.

There is no clinical evidence that you can 'spot-reduce', lose fat from a desired place, but with the right type of exercise and nutrition, you can lose the excess fat from all the problem areas. Fat loss is generally not accomplished by dieting alone. Only exercise can cause this to happen. Certain drugs and herbs can also cause fat loss, but we don't recommend those here. Losing excess fat not only makes you look better, but it also makes you healthier. Hopefully one day, measuring body fat will become as easy and straightforward

as stepping on the bathroom scales, so that this becomes the normal way of monitoring the state that we're in.

How to measure body fat

Unfortunately it is not as easy to measure body fat as it is to weigh yourself. You can get body fat measured at some doctor's surgeries and chemists, or at a health club. The caliper method is the most straightforward. Calipers measure your subcutaneous fat at certain skinfolds which have been found to correlate highly with body fat.

Body fat can also be measured by magnetic resonance imaging, weighing the body in and out of water and using the difference to calculate body fat, and bio-electric impedance which is based on the fact that electricity will pass quicker through muscle than fat. But these methods require high-tech expensive equipment.

Regardless of the method used, the number given will be a percentage. This percentage represents the per cent of your body weight which is taken up by fat. By multiplying this percentage by your total weight, you can determine how much actual fat you possess.

If you are 10 stone and 20% fat, it means that your body consists of 28 pounds of fat and 112 pounds lean body mass (bone, muscle, organ tissue, blood and everything else).

Some fat is essential for bodily functions. Fat regulates body temperature, cushions and insulates organs and tissues and is the main form of the body's energy storage.

Though there's not a recommended range in Britain, Table 1 describes body fat ranges and their associated categories.

Table 1. From American Council of Exercise. Note, due to measurement differences, American fat percentages tend to be lower than European recommendations.

Age	Risky	Excellent	Good	Fair	Poor	Very Poor
19-24	<9%	18.9%	22.1%	25.0%	29.6%	>29.6%
25-29		18.9%	22.0%	25.4%	29.8%	>29.8%
30-34		19.7%	22.7%	26.4%	30.5%	>30.5%
35-39		21.0%	24.0%	27.7%	31.5%	>31.5%
40-44		22.6%	25.6%	29.3%	32.8%	>32.8%
45-49		24.3%	27.3%	30.9%	34.1%	>34.1%
50-54		26.6%	29.7%	33.1%	36.2%	>36.2%
55-59		27.4%	30.7%	34.0%	37.3%	>37.3%
60+		27.6%	31.0%	34.4%	38.0%	>38.0%

The Science of Fat

The percentage gets higher as we get older because we naturally lose muscle as we age. Knowing your body fat percentage can help you determine if your weight loss goals are realistic for a woman of your age.

The fuels we need to live

Fat tissue is the major energy store of the body and its size can only increase if food intake is greater than the body's energy output. Thermogenesis is the generation of heat by the burning of calories. This heat, or energy output can be influenced by several things: metabolic rate, cold, and exercise.

There is also a capacity for energy release on eating, which is the thermic effect of food. Variations in any of these factors will alter energy output, and hence the amount of food that can be eaten without weight gain.

We use different types of fuel for different forms of activity:

● Protein
● Carbohydrates
● Fats

Protein is used very little for fuel. Carbohydrates and fats are our main sources of fuel for energy.

Protein is the body's chief building material. Our muscles, bones, cartilage, skin, hair and blood are all made in part from protein. A good supply of protein is essential when you are pregnant or breast feeding, and during a strength training, fat burning programme.

Carbohydrates may be simple (sugars) or complex (starches). Simple carbohydrates (sugars), found in sweets and chocolate, are high in calories and provide instant energy. When you eat sugar, your blood sugar level rises dramatically, and your pancreas releases insulin to stabilise this raised level. Your blood sugar then drops very quickly, making you feel tired and lacking energy. Too much sugar on its own in a meal or snack will cause you to gain weight, and your body cannot burn fat when insulin levels are high.

Complex carbohydrates (starches) are the real energy foods. Grains, rice, potatoes and vegetables all contain large amounts of starch. Your body has to work harder to digest starches, even harder if they are unrefined, such as wholemeal bread, wholewheat pasta and brown rice. This provides you with long-lasting energy, keeps your blood sugar level constant, and keeps your appetite satisfied for longer.

Starches can be further divided into '*fast burning*' and '*slow burning*' starches, and high and low glycaemic indexes, which are also key to efficient use of food and fat reduction. I will go into further detail in Chapter 6.

Fat is the second energy food. When you're trying to lose fat and replace it with muscle, you may think of fat as the enemy, but it's not. We all need fat in our diets, but like carbohydrates, there are fats that will make you fatter, and fats that are an essential part of a healthy diet.

Why diets don't work

The last thing that a new mother should do is go on a diet. She needs to give herself the very best nutrients to cope with the demands of caring for an infant. And if she's breast feeding, good nutrients are even more important.

An even stronger reason is that diets don't work. On most restrictive diets, very little of the weight actually lost is fat. You are more likely to lose water, lean muscle, and even bone tissue as well as fat.

Diets are short term and come to an end, and when you resort to your previous eating habits, the weight comes back as fat. This is because once you start eating less, your body, realising that its fuel supply is being restricted, goes into survival mode. It will lower its metabolism so it can function on fewer calories, and your fat cells will become more efficient at holding onto and storing fat.

Your metabolism will stay down for a long time after you stop dieting. So as soon as you stop dieting you will lay down fat because your metabolism is lower and your body is preparing itself for the next famine. Even if you just go back up to your original weight you will actually have a higher body fat content as your lost muscle has now been replaced with fat.

As the weight comes back on, you go on another diet, which repeats the cycle, and further increases your body fat. With this yo-yo dieting, you are draining yourself mentally, spiritually, physically, and emotionally. Nutritionist Tom Sanders describes dieting as the western world's answer to Chinese foot-binding: institutionalised torture of women's bodies. The only way to achieve the body you want is through healthy nutrition combined with a well designed exercise programme.

So how do you lose fat?

The best way to lose fat and keep it off, is through a programme of dietary modification and exercise. And to get the full benefit of exercise, you need to do both strength training and cardiovascular conditioning (aerobic work). As you get stronger, each pound of muscle you add will burn about 40 calories per day extra of fat.

The purpose of cardiovascular training is to actually burn calories during the exercise, which is how you achieve the calorific reduction that leads to weight loss. And the more of those calories burnt that are fat calories, the better the result.

The purpose of strength training is to maintain or even increase muscle mass. As stated earlier, the biggest problem with dieting alone is the loss of muscle tissue which leads to a decrease in metabolism. With regular strength training, this can be avoided.

An American study was conducted to compare weight loss in three groups. All groups were set up to lose a pound per week by removing 500 calories per day from their diet by various means. The first cut calories by 500 per day. The second cut calories by 250 a day and exercised to burn 250 calories a day. The third exercised to burn 500 calories a day. After 12 weeks members of all three groups had lost about 11 pounds which was to be expected. However, the difference was in the composition of the weight lost. The first group lost about 50% fat and 50% muscle, the second group lost 65-70% fat, and the third group lost about 90% of the weight as fat.

> To reduce body fat, you need to focus on increasing the amount of exercise you do, rather than decreasing the amount of food you eat.

Eating healthily to reduce fat

In the presence of carbohydrate, the preferred fuel is glucose and the capacity to mobilise fat is limited. Factors that increase blood glucose during dieting may stimulate insulin release and all the metabolic consequences of circulating insulin. Fatty acid synthesis is activated and lipolysis – or the breaking down of fat, is profoundly inhibited by insulin even at very low concentrations of the hormone[4].

These studies indicate a low carbohydrate diet with generous protein allowance provides superior fat loss, and reduced lean tissue loss compared to other types of weight loss diets. The main disadvantage is a greater incidence of tiredness, which can be countered by staying active.

Aerobic conditioning to burn fat

Aerobic conditioning can help you to burn calories and raise your metabolic rate, giving you a high from the body's 'feel good' hormones (endorphins). These are released when you exercise and give you an emotional lift. It also makes your heart work more efficiently, tones the muscles, helps you relax, decreases your stress levels, and help you sleep more soundly and deeply.

And the best type of aerobic conditioning, especially if you are a new mother, in addition to all the above benefits, is that which:
● is most efficient at burning fat
● is as intensive as you want to make it
● is least injurious to joints for even the overweight
● is enjoyable for the beginner
● you can perform regularly without fatiguing yourself
● freely accessible and cost effective
● can include partners, other family members, and most importantly, your baby.

That exercise is walking. We strongly advocate the importance of walking, which is the perfect exercise after pregnancy. It is low risk, the impact of brisk walking is only about 1.3 times your body weight, compared with high impact jogging and running which have an impact of approximately three times your body weight. It is also one of the best exercises for strengthening bones, controlling weight, toning the leg muscles, maintaining good posture and improving positive self-image. Walking also helps to slow the ageing process.

American doctor Ali Fathy is a septuagenarian, and has conducted a study of regular exercisers – male and female – over 20 years. The exercisers walked as part of their regular exercise routines. Dr Fathy compared their body fat averages with that of non-exercisers of the same age. The exercisers' body fat averaged at 20%. The non-exercisers averaged at 26%.

Walk your way to fitness

Walking is the best way to burn fat. When I first discovered this I thought it couldn't be right. Surely to burn fat efficiently the exercise has got to hurt? Thankfully, 'no pain no gain' is a complete myth. When you feel pain when doing high impact exercises what you are feeling is the effect of lactic acid on the muscles. (Lactic acid is a substance produced in the muscles when they become fatigued.) You are not burning fat. Walking is more efficient at burning fat than running, though you do use up more total calories running than walking.

The Science of Fat

A study to illustrate this point was conducted at the University of Wisconsin in the United States. A group of subjects walked on a treadmill for 30 minutes at a self-selected, comfortable walking pace. Subjects walked at an average of 3.8 mph (16 minutes per mile), and burned approximately 8 kcal per minute, and their RER value was .88, indicating that they were expending 59% of their calories from carbohydrates and 41% of their calories from fat. When asked to run for 30 minutes at a comfortable pace, subjects ran at an average of 6.5 mph (nine minutes per mile) and expended approximately 15 kcal per minute. They were expending 76% carbohydrates and 24% fat.

Running did result in a greater total calorific expenditure, and a slightly higher total number of calories from fat, but walking was more efficient at fat burning using up 41% over 30 minutes compared with 24% fat used up when running.

To lose fat, it's more important to build up time than speed. Walking at a moderate pace yields longer workouts with less soreness. You cover more distance and burn off more fat.

Pros and cons of high-intensity versus low-intensity workouts
Pros:
- High-intensity workouts burn the most calories per minute. Important if you have limited time.
- High intensity raises the body's metabolic rate for a few hours afterwards, resulting in a few more calories expended.
- Increased workout intensity usually means increased fitness levels.

Cons:
- The higher the intensity, the greater the risk of injury.
- You are more likely to cut your workouts or give up completely if you were required to do three high intensity workouts per week.
- You cannot sustain a longer workout, i.e. moderate walking can be sustained for up to two hours or even longer. High intensity workouts can only be sustained for 30-45 minutes if you're already fit. Only serious athletes can go on for longer.

Many people find low intensity more enjoyable and will therefore exercise more consistently.

Anyone can walk for fitness. You only need a pair of properly fitting athletic shoes or walking boots, and somewhere to walk – a park, shopping centre, or treadmill. Walking can be mild – where you can go on indefinitely; moderate – can

be sustained for up to two hours if you are already fairly fit, and you can talk easily; and race walking-pace which is high intensity and can only be sustained for 30-45 minutes for the already fit.

How long do you have to walk to burn fat
Many in the exercise world believe that you can walk, or do other low intensity exercise for 20 minutes, then anything over and above that 20 minutes and you are only burning fat. This is a myth. Your body burns both glycogen (carbohydrate) and stored fat during exercise. Glycogen burning is favoured during the beginning of exercise and during intense exercise. Fat burning is maximised during sustained, low intensity exercise. The longer you work out the more exhausted your supply of glycogen becomes and the more fat your body burns.

But though you are burning more fat after 20 minutes, you are not burning only fat. The body always uses a combination of fat and carbohydrate during exercise.

Moderate-intensity, long duration (20-60 minutes) walking is ideal for fat loss. And it is logical that the longer you walk, the more fat you will lose, and if you get into a regular routine, you will maximise fat loss. But it is incorrect to think that there's a magic fat burning device that comes on after 20 minutes.

Walking technique
Talking about a technique for walking may seem like a way to complicate the easiest of activities. But adding a little technique to your stride will make things feel easier, and less of a grind, and make your walks more efficient in burning fat. A few useful tips are:
- Swing your arms in a controlled manner. Bend arms a little at the elbow to make a shorter, faster swing which will in turn make your legs move faster because arms and legs have to move in unison.
- Don't take long, exaggerated strides in an attempt to move faster.
- Push off with your rear toe. Your rear leg should lengthen, and your toes are the last thing to leave the ground. You should feel the ball of your foot push into the ground causing a reaction that propels you forward.
- Strike on the heel of your other foot as you land, and allow the ankle to move through its full range of motion.
- Think of walking from your waist, allowing each hip bone to extend forward with it's respective leg. You'll feel a slight rotation in the lower back that allows the leg to swing more freely while each stride can cover more ground and you move faster.

Treadmills

If the weather is bad, or walking outside doesn't suit you, you could invest in a treadmill or use one at a health club or gym. Walking on a treadmill gives you the same fat burning benefits as walking outdoors, but more versatility. The same technique rules apply. You do walk slightly differently on a treadmill because the belt rotating underneath your feet means you're doing tiny jumps up and down as you walk instead of just pushing off from behind. And the belt may cause you to slap down your front foot harder than usual which could put additional pressure on your shins.

Do not walk on an inclined treadmill when pregnant this increases the pressure on your back. If you're thinking of buying a treadmill, you have to be prepared to spend at least £500 on a motorised one. Don't buy an un-motorised treadmill just because it is cheaper, they are a strain on the joints, and they alter your technique because you are forced to push and pull the belt along.

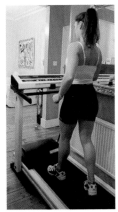

Look for:

- wide rubber treads
- a minimum 1.5 horsepower
- controls that are easy to operate
- a safety catch so that children cannot start the machine
- a panic shut-off in case you get into difficulty.
- a hand rail for balance
- a top speed of 10 miles per hour
- inclines of up to 15%.

TEST THE TREADMILL BEFORE YOU BUY IT.

References

1. *Journal of Paediatric Medicine* (1981) 98:883-87.
2. *American Journal of Clinical Nutrition* (1993) 57:140-45.
3. McArdle *et al. Essentials of Exercise Physiology,* p.485.
4. *American Journal of Clinical Nutrition* (1992) 57:217-23.

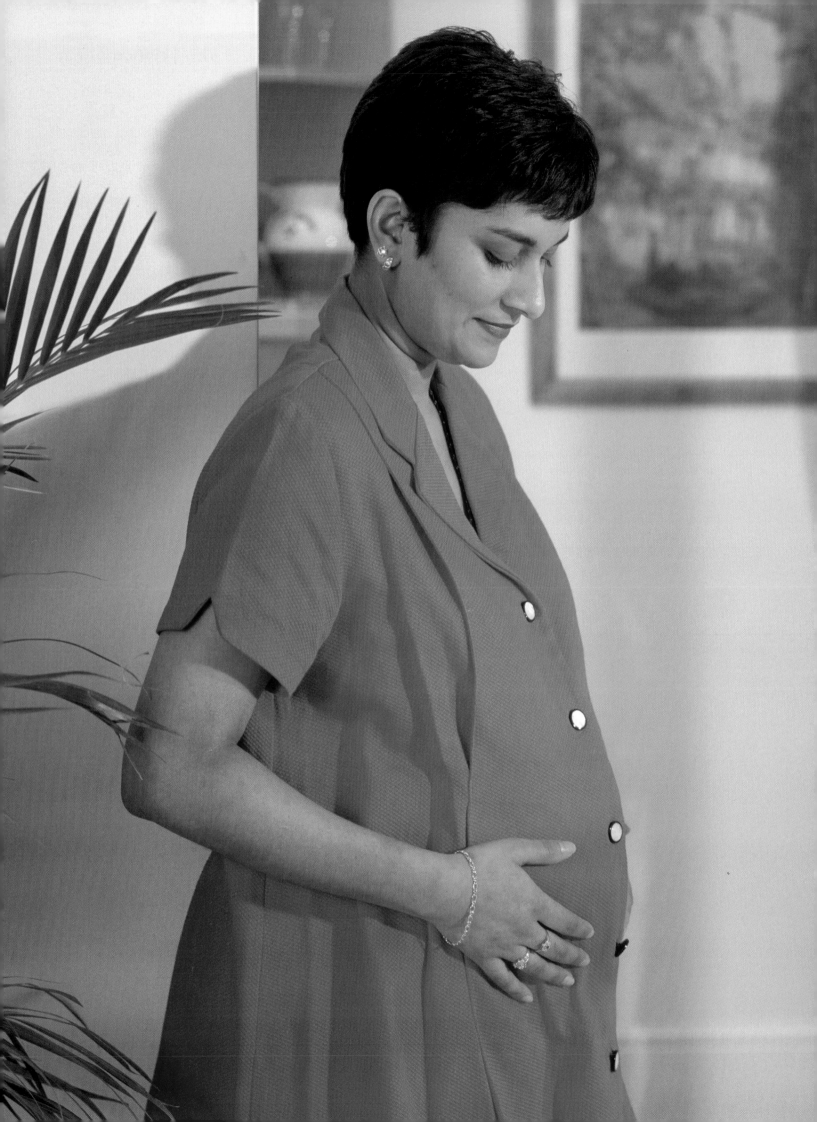

Positive Pregnancy

Your body goes through many physiological and emotional changes while you are pregnant. Understanding the changes can help you prepare for them in a positive way. Where things start to get uncomfortable, we have a wealth of suggestions for minimising the discomfort.

Professor Craig Sharp has described pregnancy as 'progressive resistance training'. In other words, your body will naturally achieve in pregnancy, the physiological benefits that professional endurance athletes take years of training to achieve.

Professor Sharp has extensively studied the fitness of pregnant women. In one study, 12 women who were two to three months pregnant, and at different levels of fitness ranging from unfit to very fit, took a series of fitness tests. Professor Sharp tested their level of fitness, then after doing no exercise at all, he tested their fitness levels two to three weeks after giving birth. He found that the very fit women were less fit than before their pregnancies, the moderately fit showed no change, and the unfit women were considerably fitter after their pregnancies.

The main reason for this is the most striking physiological change that occurs during pregnancy – the increase in your blood volume.

Blood volume
The level of increase in your blood volume varies according to your age, size, number of pregnancies, and whether you are having one baby or a multiple birth. The average increase in blood volume is 30-45%. Extra blood is needed to carry the oxygen and nutrients to nourish the fetus, and your organs, especially the kidneys, are working harder. If you exercise during and after your pregnancy, you can maximise the positive effect of the increased blood volume transporting more oxygen to feed the muscles. This is what top athletes strive for.

Hormone activity
Over 30 hormones control and instigate the physiological changes in pregnancy. These are the most important:

Progesterone is the main hormone of pregnancy. It is initially produced by the ovaries, until the placenta takes over. Progesterone relaxes the smooth muscle of the uterus, stomach, bowels, and bladder, stimulates glandular tissue in the breasts, and raises body temperature.

Oestrogen stimulates the growth of the uterus, increases the size of the nipples, and primes the uterus to contract at the onset of labour.

Relaxin loosens the pubic symphysis joint of the pelvic floor to make room for the birth of the child.

Aldosterone controls the body's salt and water balance to allow the increase in blood volume.

Thyroid stimulating hormone (TSH) regulates metabolism.

Parathyroid hormone (PTH) controls the metabolism of calcium, phosphorus and magnesium.

Growth hormone helps the body to develop muscle tissue. So while a large proportion of added weight is fat, you are also developing lean muscle.

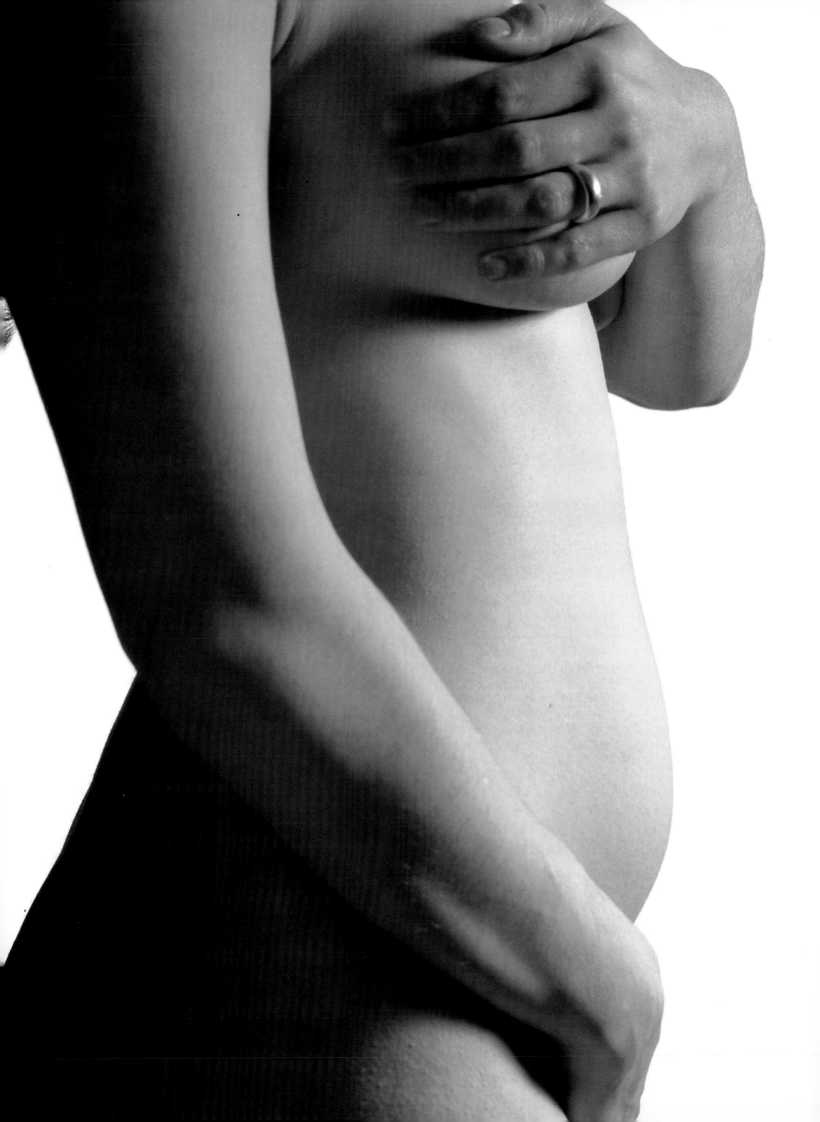

First trimester

(conception to 3 months)
As soon as you conceive, your body is programmed to undergo a precisely planned series of natural changes and adjustments which prepare it to create and nurture a new life. The ovum implants into the uterus wall, triggering hormonal changes. Increased levels of oestrogen and progesterone switch on a highly efficient signalling system which ensures that your body adapts to provide the ideal environment for your baby's development.

By the time you miss a period, crucial changes have already taken place, and the embryo has already reached a vital phase of growth. This hormone activity is reflected in early pregnancy symptoms, such as breast discomfort, tiredness, urinating more frequently and for some a tendency to be more emotional than usual.

Women do not all experience pregnancy in the same way. The most common complaints during the first trimester are fatigue, nausea and vomiting. Some women have severe nausea and vomiting, while others get through without any queasiness. While sickness causes some women to lose their appetites, many others begin to have an increased appetite by the third month.

Most women experience breast changes. At first the breasts become tender. As the trimester continues, the breasts often become heavier and the areola (the pigmented area around the nipple) darkens. During the whole pregnancy, breasts may increase in size and weight by up to 40%.

Indigestion, bloating, and flatulence are common. Some women tend to become constipated because the hormones of pregnancy slow digestion. Many women find that they sweat more.

Despite all these symptoms, most women do not show much during the first trimester. Total weight gain is typically only two or three pounds. However, by the end of the trimester, you may have a small swelling above the pubic bone.

Second trimester

(4 months to 6 months)
The second trimester is a time of rapid growth for the mother and baby. In this period, a woman gains about a pound a week. The uterus grows to the navel by the end of this trimester. The pregnancy is now obvious to the mother

and others. For most women, nausea generally subsides early in the trimester. Most women gain energy, and some have that radiance or glow of pregnancy. Most women have a healthy appetite, and some experience food cravings.

By about 20 weeks (24-26 if it's a first pregnancy), most women can feel their baby moving. By the sixth month, a woman may notice occasional tightenings and relaxation of the uterus. These non-rhythmic contractions, called Braxton-Hicks, are normal. They help the uterus prepare for labour. Rhythmic contractions which become increasingly frequent and painful are not normal and may indicate premature labour.

The breasts grow, as does the abdomen. Veins appear on the breasts and the areolae continue to darken. A dark line, the linea nigra, may appear between the navel and the pubis. This will fade after birth. A thin, white vaginal discharge is normal. Other complaints may include heartburn, wind, constipation, dizziness and fainting, swollen feet, haemorrhoids, muscle cramps, varicose veins and backache.

Third trimester

(6 months to birth)
The abdomen grows rapidly in the third trimester. As the months progress, the uterus comes close to the ribcage, which often causes breathlessness. At around seven months it is possible to see the baby's movements through the mother's abdomen. During this trimester, a pregnant woman will experience more Braxton-Hicks contractions in preparation for labour.

Most women feel awkward during this trimester as their large abdomen shifts their natural balance. The last days of pregnancy may be quite uncomfortable. The rapidly growing baby crowds the abdomen and puts stress on the back. As in the second trimester, heartburn, constipation, and haemorrhoids are common. Frequent urination results from the uterus pressing on the bladder, and fatigue returns. Backache, muscle cramps, and swelling of the hands and feet are common. Vaginal discharge increases, and some women begin to leak colostrum (the beginning of breast milk) from their nipples.

Skin changes
In the first trimester, your skin can become dry and sensitive. During the second, the subtle changes become even

Positive Pregnancy

4

more evident as your skin becomes taut and stretched to accommodate your growing baby. Hormones begin to naturally break down the collagen and elastin tissues, causing your skin to look and feel dry, irritated, uncomfortably stretched and thin.

The third trimester brings even more dramatic change as you lose sight of your feet somewhere below your belly. On average, a pregnant woman's skin stretches from 17 square feet to 18.5 square feet by the time she's ready to deliver. Because the skin stretches so much during pregnancy, many women get stretch marks (striae). The exact cause is not clear, but many believe that they are scars within the dermis caused when the collagen in the skin ruptures leaving gaps.

They are very difficult to get rid of, but you can help prevent them by feeding your skin from the inside by good nutrition, and from the outside by nourishing oils (see page 81).

Changes in skin pigmentation, called chloasma, are common on the face during pregnancy. Up to three in four women may develop these changes. The changes are characterised by a blotchy brown increase in pigment. Several factors are involved in the development of chloasma including race, sun exposure and hormones (both oestrogen and progesterone stimulate pigment formation).

Weight gain and fat deposition
During pregnancy, fat is deposited on the breasts, hips, bottom, thighs, and upper arms. This fat is an important insulator and energy store, especially when breast feeding.

Table 2. Accepted weight gain during pregnancy is 25-35 lbs. This can be broken down into:

Substance	Weight (pounds)
Fetus	7.5
Fat, protein and other nutrients (including breast growth)	9
Increased blood and fluid	8
Uterus	2
Amniotic fluid	2
Placenta	1.5
Total	30

Emotional changes
Pregnancy is a time of adjustment and emotional swings are quite normal. Understanding the physical and emotional changes of pregnancy may help to make your pregnancy a positive experience.

First trimester
In the first trimester, you may find that your emotions are unstable and that you feel depressed for no apparent reason. It is commonly believed that the mood changes in pregnancy are caused by hormonal changes.

You may have mixed feelings about your pregnancy and the changes it will bring. You will naturally feel anxious about the safety of your baby during your pregnancy, labour and delivery.

Second trimester
The highlight of the second trimester is feeling the baby move. The growing abdomen and fetal movements make the pregnancy seem real. Other people notice the pregnancy, and the attention can make you feel quite special.

You may now perceive the baby as a real person and become more excited about the pregnancy. Women sometimes have more energy and feel better during the second trimester, commonly known as the 'glow' of pregnancy. Endorphins steadily rise till about the middle of the second trimester, then they gradually fall. At this peak, they may be over five times higher than the levels found in athletes who claim to feel the 'runners high'.

Third trimester
The third trimester combines a sense of pride with anxiety about the birth. During the final weeks you may feel more anxious and more uncomfortable. Often, women fear that something may be wrong with the baby. You may not be able to find a comfortable position to sleep.
Women are eager for the discomforts of pregnancy to end, but also concerned about the reality of becoming a mother and the changes in marital and family relationships. The prospect of pain in labour, especially if it is a first pregnancy, can be daunting.

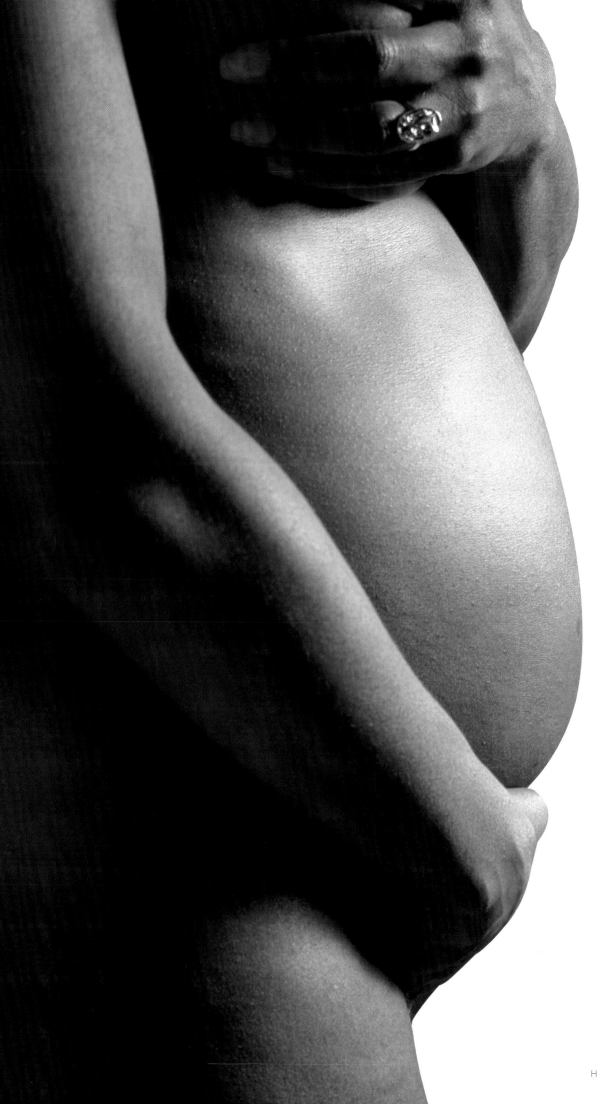

4

Advice for positive labour

- Be as prepared as you can be by attending ante-natal classes and reading books and magazines.

- Speak to women who have had babies. Ask them honestly about their experiences, but remember that your experience will be unique to you.

- Write a birth plan, but don't be too rigid about the type of birth that you want. Be flexible about pain relief, and find out what is available. For example, not all hospitals have an anaesthetist available 24 hours a day to administer epidurals.

- Try to take your birth partner with you to ante-natal classes, so that he or she knows what you want and can take over or speak on your behalf.

- You can ask for a different midwife during delivery if you feel that you are not getting the support you need.

- If your birth experience is traumatic, seek help from your health visitor, GP or a counsellor.

ALTERNATIVE REMEDIES FOR PREGNANCY PROBLEMS

Nausea

Morning sickness or nausea can be the worst thing about pregnancy. Some women have a very mild form in early pregnancy, while others suffer terribly all the way through. Until you have it, you won't come anywhere near under-standing how bad it can be. I'm told seasickness comes close, but for me, it meant not feeling human until the sixth month of pregnancy. I felt that my body had been taken over by an alien, and in a way it had. About 75-80% of pregnant women get it, and not just in the morning.

Nausea is thought to be caused by the many physiological and biochemical changes taking place inside the body. These changes include rapidly increasing oestrogen levels, an enhanced sense of smell, excess stomach acids, and increased fatigue. It may also be associated with the depth of implantation of the conceptus in the uterus, so at least nausea may imply a lower risk of miscarriage.

How to relieve nausea

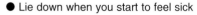
- Lie down when you start to feel sick
- Avoid getting overtired get lots of rest

Key to icons
In the next sections the icons below are used to highlight suggestions in the text

 Common sense

 Diet

 Homeopathy

 Oils

 Exercise

 Medical

- Make a note of things that trigger nausea so that you can avoid them; odours, and sudden motion can be triggers

- Eat frequent small meals that contain some carbohydrate and protein
- Drink plenty of water between meals
- Eat something every one to two hours
- Keep a drink and a dry biscuit like a ryvita or an oatcake by your bed. When you wake up, eat the biscuit before you lift your head. Sit up very slowly and have your drink. Then rest for about 20 minutes before you get out of bed
- Avoid rich, fatty, spicy, acidic or fried foods, and foods laden with preservatives and additives
- Ask yourself what will make you feel better: something crunchy, salty, sour, fruity or sweet? Eat it. Don't worry about perfect nutrition right now
- Try 50-100 mg, vitamin B6 twice a day
- Discontinue taking your usual vitamins for a few days, then reintroduce them gradually
- Sip peppermint, raspberry leaf, anise or fennel tea
- Ginger tea may be helpful: grate some ginger into a cup, pour hot water on it and add a little honey to taste.
- Or try sucking candied ginger

- Try a dropperful of wild yam tincture in a glass of water, or, HomIpecac, nux vomica, or Sepia 6c (see a home-opath for further advice)

- Use acupressure. Look at your wrist on the palm side. Locate the crease furthest from your hand between your hand and wrist. Measure two thumb widths up from this crease, and press in the middle of your wrist at this spot. There is an acupressure point here. If you stimulate for several seconds, you may help to relieve nausea and motion sickness it works for many people. If you have the point, you should feel a distinct twinge when you stimulate it. You may use it several times a day. Sea Bands are soft cotton wristbands with a plastic button that pushes against the acupressure point in your wrist. They can help stave off nausea
- Relaxation, visualisation, or self-hypnosis may help

- The smell of lemons seems to help. Sniff a cut lemon, burn lemon oil in your bedroom at night or put two drops of lemon oil on a handkerchief and inhale it when you feel queasy.

- Speak to your doctor if you vomit so often that you can not keep any food down. Excessive vomiting in pregnancy (hyperemesis gravidarium) is rare, but if you don't treat it you can become malnourished and dehydrated, which is dangerous for you and your baby
- Do not take any medication, including vitamins, herbal or homeopathic remedies without first contacting your midwife, doctor or accredited practitioner.

How pregnancy affects a woman's ability to exercise

Change	Effect on Exercise	What we recommend
The respiratory rate is naturally increased, the functional capacity of the lungs decreases by 25% and the diaphragm elevates. The heart works harder to give enough oxygen to the developing fetus.	Can reduce the amount of oxygen available for exercise.	Avoid strenuous aerobic exercises that make you breathless.
The womb enlarges, the lower back develops more curvature, and your centre of gravity shifts.	Changes your sense of balance, and requires adjustments in posture to prevent injury.	Avoid exercises that can cause loss of balance and exercises that involve lying on your back after the first trimester.
The body produces a hormone called relaxin.	Relaxin loosens the joints of the pelvis to make room for the baby to pass through the birth canal. But because all of the joints in the body become more lax, there is a greater chance of spraining.	Avoid exercises that strain joints or overstretch muscles. Especially avoid carrying heavy shopping bags with your arms extended down your sides as this can lead to sore wrists, elbows and shoulders.
During pregnancy your body metabolises carbohydrates more quickly. Exercise also increases the metabolism of carbohydrates.	These two factors can lead to low blood sugar reactions during exercise.	Eat more slow burning carbohydrates (see Chapter 6).
Your blood volume increases by about 40%, and your heart rate by about 15 beats per minute.	The flow of blood in the body can be disrupted	Avoid exercising for long periods of time
Increased blood flow to the skin.	Helps to cool the body.	Avoid exercise that makes you too hot.

Positive Pregnancy

Breast discomfort

One of the first signs of pregnancy is enlarged or sore breasts. After pregnancy, many women complain of breast sagging.

 It is important to wear a well-fitting bra with firm straps, day and night, and change sizes regularly. Do not wear under-wired bras they can press on the milk ducts and cause blockages.

 Do chest exercises (see pages 104 and 117) to tone the pectoral muscles which support your breasts.

 Massage your breasts day and night with jojoba or wheat-germ oil, or this mixture: to 4 tablespoons of almond oil, add 7 drops of mandarin or tangerine oil and 5 drops of neroli oil.

Sleep and fatigue

Being pregnant will make you feel tired, and later on in your pregnancy you may find it difficult to get to sleep. The most important thing to do is to listen to your body, be honest with yourself if you have been over working, and slow down.

How to energise yourself during pregnancy

● Take naps. Even closing your eyes for 15 minutes and letting yourself drift off can help.
● Try to vary your daily routine as boredom can be exhausting and try to do some gentle exercise.
● Try to do as many household chores as you can sitting down, for example, ironing and preparing food. Better still, try and get someone else to do them!

● Eat well from a wide range of foods especially protein
● Eat frequently. Smaller, more frequent meals can give you more energy.
● Eat energy boosting foods for lunch, such as slow burning carbohydrates (see page 64). During pregnancy your body uses carbohydrates more quickly.

● Try alternating kali phosphoricum and calcarea phosphoricum (doses)

● To a warm (not hot) bath, add 2 drops of lavender oil, 1 drop of mandarin oil and 1 drop of ylang ylang oil. Relax for at least 10 minutes.

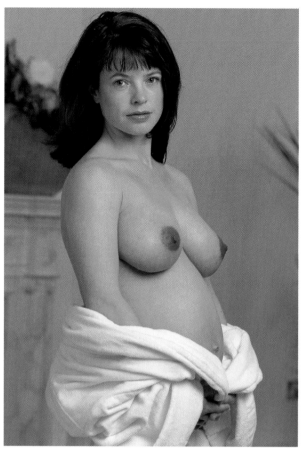

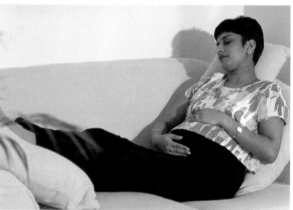

During the third trimester the ideal position for sleep is on the left side. You may find it helpful to prop your upper leg and abdomen on pillows. This allows maximum blood flow to the placenta, better kidney function, and improved blood return to the heart. Sleeping on the back is not recommended the weight of the womb constricts blood flow and can impair digestion and breathing.

Anaemia

You may be tired because you are anaemic and need to increase the amount of iron in your diet (see page 69), and take a supplement.

Take a herbal iron tonic which you can buy at your health food store. If this does not suit you, try a low potency of Ferrum Metallicum with Calearea Phosphoricum to stimulate the body to absorb iron more effectively. Also drink fresh orange (or any citrus) juice with your meals as this aids the absorption of iron, and drink nettle tea as this is high in iron.

Posture

Having a large amount of weight in front of you when you are heavily pregnant can badly affect your posture. Exercise can help, and you should be aware of your posture all the time (see page 80).

Always be aware of your back. Whether you are driving in a car, or sitting in a chair with a high back, remember to push your navel back towards your spine, and hold torso upright. If you have an office job, or work at a computer or telephone, remember not to slouch your shoulders and round your back. When you are sitting, your knees should always be higher than your bottom, and your back straight. You could rest your feet on a telephone directory.

Do not stand for long periods of time. If you cannot avoid this, check that your abdominals are pulled in, and your hips are slightly tucked under with your knees relaxed. Wearing high heels can cause you to arch your back, which can result in back pain and fatigue. If you like the extra height, wedge heels are better.

Keep checking your posture throughout the day, or whenever you see a mirror or your reflection.

Strength training for the shoulders (see page 106) and exercises that retract the shoulder blades and stretch the chest (see page 107) will help your posture.

There is anecdotal evidence that good posture can lead to easier labour. When the baby is in the right position, labour is easier. The secret of optimal fetal positioning is good posture.

Postural changes in pregnancy – and how exercise can help

Change taking place	How exercise can help
Stretching and thinning of the abdominal wall often contributes to low back pain and discomfort.	Strengthens the abdominal and lower back muscles to minimise postural changes and lower back pain.
The centre of gravity shifts forward, and the pelvis also rotates forward.	Increases muscle tone in all muscle groups to minimise postural changes.
Your co-ordination, and balance are altered.	Strengthens the body and increases fitness to give you a greater feeling of control.
The round ligaments extend outwards from the uterus on either side of the wall of the pelvis. As the uterus enlarges, more strain is exerted on these ligaments and you may feel a sharp pain or 'stitch' that runs from the lower abdomen into the groin or upper thigh.	Pelvic tilting on hands and knees allows the uterus to relax forward out of the pelvis and the ligaments to relax. This should relieve the stitch immediately though you may look a bit funny doing this in the office.
The uterosacral ligaments extend backward from the cervix to the sacrum. If they are stretched suddenly, you may feel short, sharp pains in your lower back.	Pelvic tilts and tightening the abdominal muscles will help to relieve this discomfort.
The risk of blood clotting increases during pregnancy, and you are more likely to develop varicose veins.	Assists blood flow in the legs and feet.
The constant pressure on the pelvic floor during pregnancy can cause it to become weakened, and after birth even injured. This may lead to ineffective support of the pelvic organs, bladder leakage, and reduced sensation during lovemaking.	Pelvic floor exercises during and after pregnancy will help. Stronger muscles will heal much faster after the stretching that occurs during childbirth.

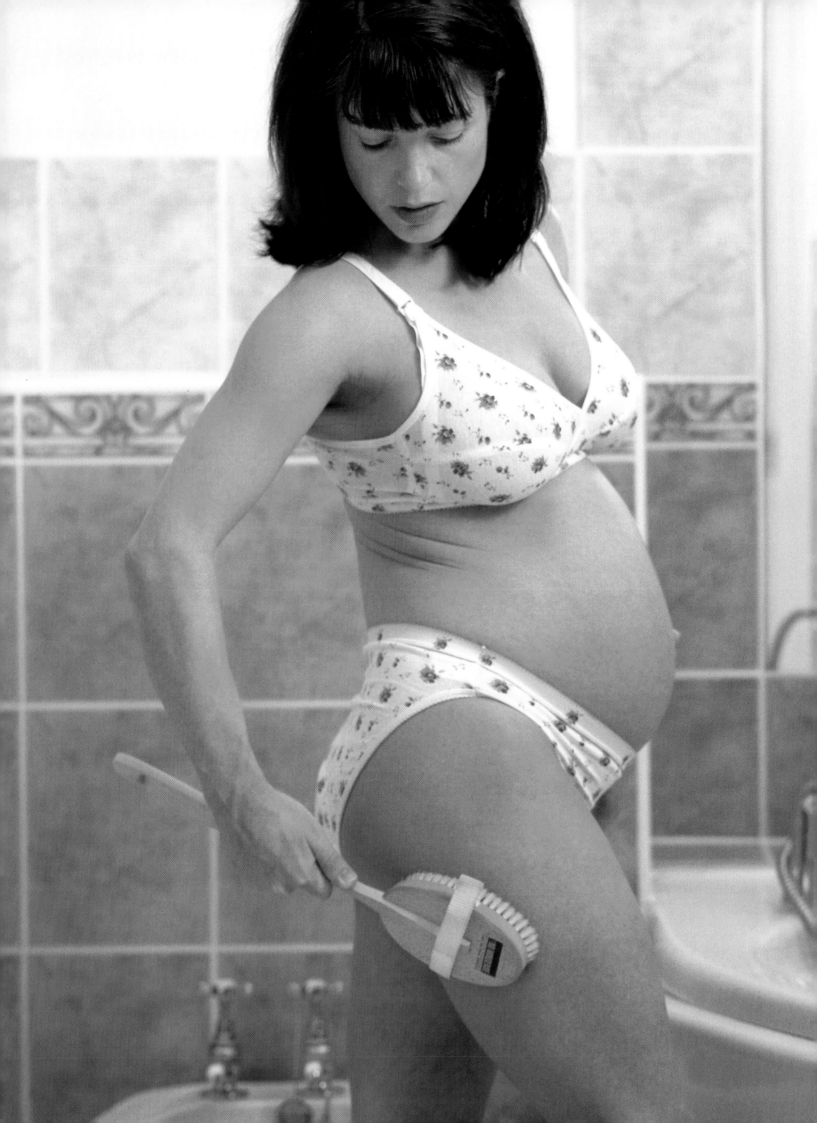

Cramp

During a cramp attack, don't stretch your leg out with your toes pointed. Instead, rub your calf and pull your foot up towards you, then hang on to the foot until the pain passes. As your pregnancy progresses, you will have to do this sitting down with legs bent.

The best way to maintain good circulation and prevent cramps is to take exercise. Our strength training programme will help tremendously, and some walking will also be beneficial.

Calcium is thought to help cramp, so eat plenty of calcium rich foods.

Try alternating between the homeopathic remedies magnesia phosphorica and calcarea phosphorica. Stop and start as needed if cramp is your only symptom.

Dry body brushing is a good way to maintain good circulation. It helps to cleanse the body of unreleased toxins. It stimulates the circulation and the lymphatic systems, encouraging the body's elimination systems to release waste.

Body brushing needs to be done every day before a bath, preferably in the morning; as in the evening it may be too stimulating and you may find you can't sleep.

How to brush your skin

- Always brush towards, and never away from your heart.
- Brush with long, firm strokes using a long-handled brush. (If the brush is scratchy at first, soaking overnight will help soften the bristles. Always remember to wash it frequently.)
- Brush very gently to begin with.
- Do one leg at time, starting at the soles of your feet (you may need some help!). Brush these and then brush over your foot, up to your knee and all around your leg. Continue up your knee, along your thigh to the buttocks, where you can brush in circular movements and a little harder.
- Brush your arms, starting at your hands and between each finger, working from the wrist to elbow and then up to your shoulder.
- Then brush your neck and back
- Avoid the breasts, but brush the chest. Go a little more slowly and gently over your trunk and abdomen, working around the lower abdomen in a clockwise direction (this is the way the large bowel goes).

After you have had your baby, we do not recommend that you body brush during the early days of breastfeeding. Skin brushing is a very stimulating treatment and will encourage the body to leak milk.

To 1¹/₂ tablespoons of almond oil add 2 drops of lavender and 2 drops of geranium oil. Mix well and use as a massage oil.

Cystitis

Urinary tract infections occur in pregnancy partly because of the pressure of the growing uterus.

Drink plenty of water to flush your system (even if you have to urinate more often this is better for you than not drinking). Or you can make your own barley water by simmering a handful of organic barley in a pint of water with a whole lemon cut in. Strain and drink. Cranberry juice is known to combat the bacteria that cause cystitis.

A sitz bath is a home made bidet. You fill a bowl with warm (not hot) water, add essential oils, and sit in it for the recommended time. For cystitis add 2 drops of lavender, sandalwood, bergamot or camomile oil. Mix well into the water and soak in it for about 5-10 minutes.

If left untreated, cystitis can develop into a serious kidney infection so always consult your doctor.

Thrush

The acid/alkaline balance of the vagina changes during pregnancy, and thrush infection is another common complaint. Vaginal discharges can become heavier, smell different and be mildly irritating.

Try to eat live natural yoghurt to help restore the 'friendly' bacteria in your intestines. It also helps to insert some yoghurt into your vagina this is very soothing. Never use bubble bath or soap if you have thrush their alkaline nature may aggravate the condition.

In a 10ml dropper bottle mix 8ml of tea tree oil and 2 drops of lavender oil. Add 2 to 4 drops of this in the bath and soak for at least 10 minutes.

Heartburn

This tends to get worse as the pregnancy progresses, before the baby's head moves down to engage in the pelvis.

Positive Pregnancy

Try to relax before you sit down to eat. Prop your pillows up when you sleep so that you are not lying flat this prevents acid leaking into the oesophagus.

Eat smaller meals and chew well as saliva aids digestion.

To ¹/₂ tablespoon of almond (or any carrier oil) add 2 drops of sandalwood oil. Use to gently massage your solar plexus, between your breasts and your bump.

Oedema (fluid retention)
This is a common pregnancy complaint, especially in the final months, though you should see your doctor if you suspect that you have excessive swelling.

The best thing is to do the exercises in Chapter 8. When you are resting, put your feet up as high as possible

If oedema is your only symptom take a short course of natrum muriaticum or apis mellifica.

Make up a massage lotion from 1¹/₂ tablespoons almond oil to which you add 2 drops of lavender oil and 2 drops of geranium oil. Ask someone to massage your legs with this oil, starting at the ankles in upward strokes to the thighs.

Haemorrhoids
These are varicose veins of the anus. The discomfort they cause can range from a slight itch to intense pain. They may also bleed, sometimes quite a lot.

Try not to strain for a bowel movement as this may cause piles.

Diet Increase the fibre and roughage in your diet to keep your bowels moving and your stools soft. Take a natural laxative such as oat bran or prunes at the first signs of constipation.

Take a warm sitz bath (see page 47) to which you have added 2 drops of geranium oil and 2 drops of cypress oil. Soak in it for 10 minutes. Or soak a pad of cotton wool in the same solution and hold it against your anus (you may find it easier to do this while sitting on the toilet). Make up a gel from 50ml of aloe gel, to which you add 5 drops of cypress oil and 5 drops of geranium oil. Mix well. Apply a small amount of this gel after you open your bowels or whenever you feel sore and itchy.

The perineum
The perineum is the skin between the vagina and the anus. It will be stretched a lot during your labour, so it is a good to moisturise it from about five months. Rub about ¹/₄ teaspoon of jojoba oil on the area. Jojoba is highly lubricating and helps the skin to be more supple. If you cannot get jojoba oil, try olive oil.

Stretch marks

By doing the exercises in the book, walking and eating well, you are already preventing stretch marks. By keeping yourself healthy you are keeping your skin healthy.

Remember to drink lots of pure fluids to keep yourself hydrated. Zinc and vitamin B6 are necessary for the health of collagen tissue, and for the maintenance of a high level of elasticity in the skin.

Try calearea gaorica, but do not take it continuously. If you have dry skin and are prone to stretch marks, take it for regular short courses throughout your pregnancy.

Pure Jojoba oil, or to 4 tablespoons of almond oil, add 7 drops of mandarin or tangerine oil and 5 drops of neroli oil. Massage into your abdomen morning and night.

Varicose veins
Varicose veins tend to develop in later pregnancy. Increased weight hinders the return of blood to the legs and can cause aching legs and throbbing pains. They can be brought on by pregnancy but they tend to disappear quite soon after.

Try not to stand still or sit with your legs crossed. The best thing you can do is exercise to help your circulation and put your feet up when you are sitting down. Try to exercise your calf muscles by flexing your feet up and down and rotating your ankle.

Make up a cooling lotion. To 100ml of unperfumed lotion, add 5 drops of geranium oil, 5 drops of lemon oil and 5 drops of cypress oil. Mix well and keep lotion in the fridge. Use to massage your legs, stroking upwards.

Overdue
If you go past the expected date of delivery your doctor or midwife may offer to induce you (start your labour artificially). But this can lead to a cascade of interventions including more pain relief, continuous monitoring and assisted (forceps, ventouse or even caesarean) delivery.

The old wives' tale about sex inducing labour has some truth to it sperm contains hormones called prostaglandins which ripen the cervix. Stimulating the nipples releases oxytocin, the hormone you produce in labour to keep contractions regular. From about the 37th week of pregnancy, stimulate one nipple at a time, rolling it gently between your thumb and forefinger for a few minutes.

Being fit and active can also kick start your labour, but be careful not to exhaust yourself.

A natural way to ripen your cervix making it softer and able to stretch more easily, is to drink raspberry leaf tea. Start at about 28 weeks with one cup a day, increase to two about three weeks later and by 37 weeks you will be drinking three cups a day. Make sure you are drinking pure raspberry leaf and not just raspberry flavoured tea. Sweeten it with honey if you need to. There is also the belief that spicy food can induce labour, and many women can testify that a curry got things going for them.

If you are late and you are offered an induction try homeopathic remedies first. Try caulophyllum, argentum nitricum, or lycopodium.

The birth

During the birth your emotions can be deep, strong and unexpected. Try aconite for anxiety, fear and panic. Arnica helps the body recover, and prevents it from going into stress.

You can burn essential oils or ask your partner to massage you with them.

Good oils:
- Rose regulates, tones and cleanses the uterus and has antidepressant qualities .
- Neroli reduces fear, apprehension and anxiety. It also helps you to breathe properly.
- Jasmine can help to dull uterine pain. It strengthens contractions, which in turn can help to shorten labour.

There are also good massage movements that you can ask your birth partner to use and it's a good idea to practise them before the big day. They press the heel of their hand into your lower back and make deep circular movements. They can also press hard in the centre of each buttock with their thumbs, pressing and releasing several times.

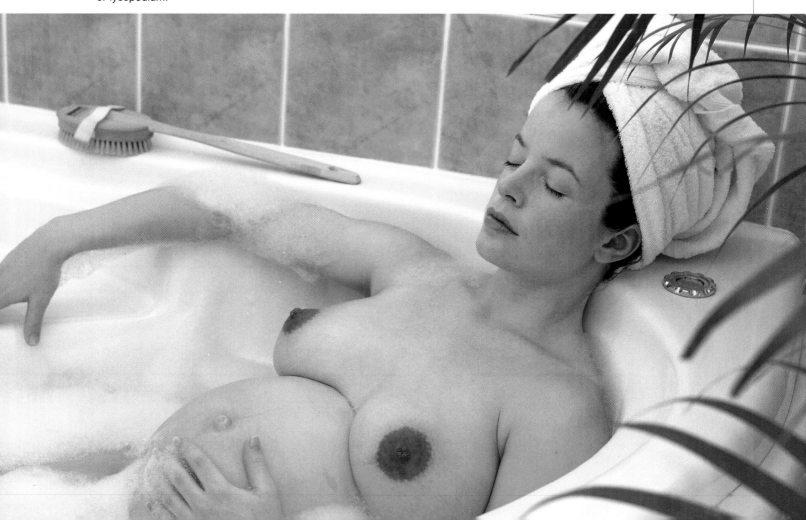

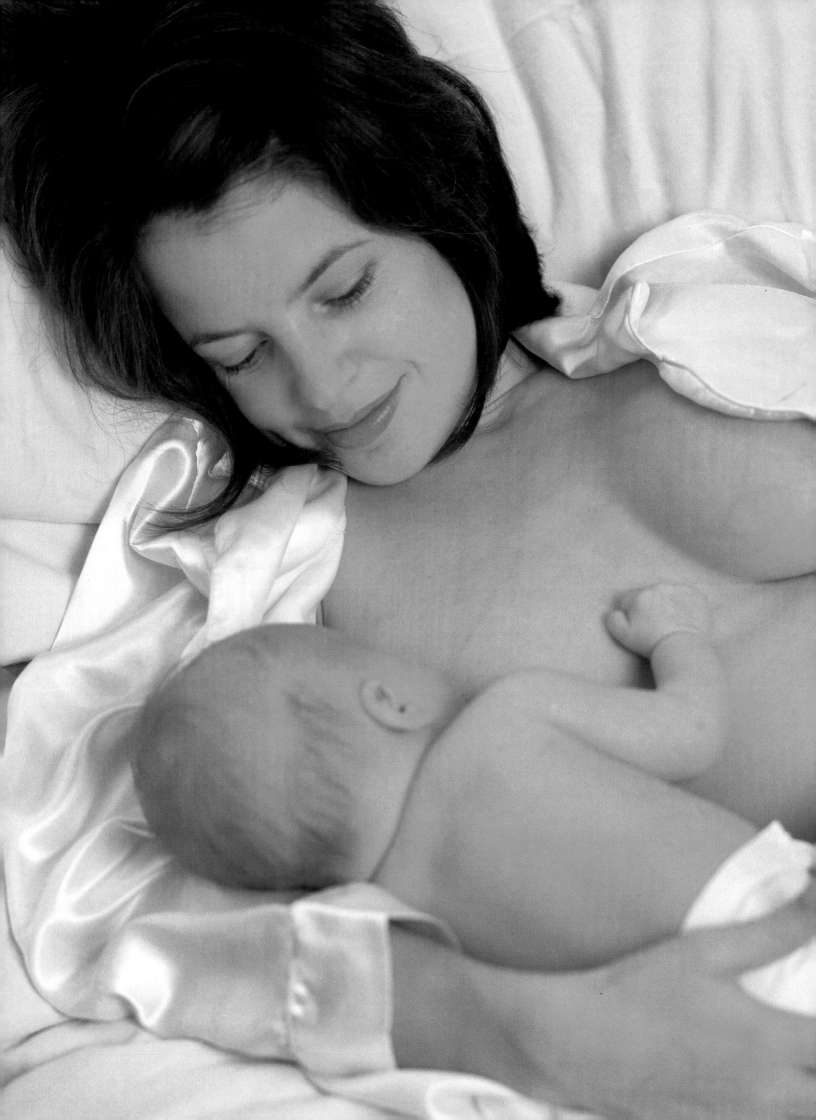

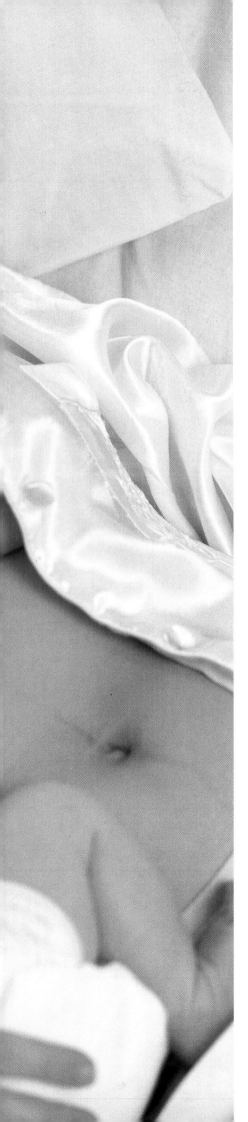

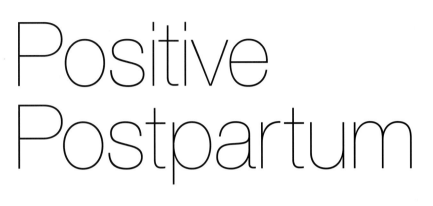

Positive Postpartum

At first, the joy of your new baby banishes any thoughts about weight or appearance, but you will soon want your body back. You can work with the changes that are going on to achieve this. But this takes discipline at a time in your life when you may feel unable to commit yourself. Because of the many changes physical and emotional that motherhood brings, it is easy to become sedentary and to lose interest in your appearance.

There is no scientific evidence that the body is predisposed to burn fat after giving birth, but there is plenty of anecdotal evidence. We understand the tremendous changes that your body has gone through over the last nine months. Our programme is all about working with your body, at your own pace, to get back into shape, not enforcing a routine for which you may not be ready. All women are different it may take you nine weeks or nine months to get back into shape. Your body is the boss, work with it.

Physiological changes

Fluid loss

The rapid weight loss of the first few weeks after childbirth is mostly loss of fluid. Around two to three litres of excess fluid is retained during pregnancy, so you can expect to make frequent trips to the lavatory to get rid of this fluid. You may also lose fluid by sweating, particularly as you sleep.

Oxytocin

The hormone oxytocin causes your uterus to contract. It takes four to six weeks to return to its pre-pregnant size. As the muscles contract you may experience 'after pains', especially during breast feeding. They usually get worse with each subsequent pregnancy.

Lochia

You will bleed for some time after birth. This is like a heavy period. From about 10 days onwards this discharge (called lochia) will change from red, to dark brown, to a whitish colour which may last for up to six weeks. If this discharge has a foul odour, tell your doctor.

Positive Postpartum

Pelvic floor

If you had a vaginal delivery, your vagina will have been left swollen, bruised and stretched. The pelvic floor muscles will also have been severely stretched, and it is not uncommon for some women to lose control of the flow of urine and leak when they cough or laugh. The pelvic floor exercises described on page 84 will help you tighten and regain tone in your vagina and pelvic floor. You can restart your pelvic floor exercises from 12 hours after your baby's birth. If you had a caesarean section, wait until you feel a bit less sore (one to two weeks). Continue doing pelvic floor exercises hourly.

Breasts

Your breasts will enlarge dramatically as they engorge (fill with milk). During the first five days after delivery you will produce colostrum, a thin white liquid which is high in protein and minerals, and low in fat and sugar. Colostrum gives your baby vital nourishment before your milk flows. Antibodies in colostrum are believed to increase your baby's resistance to disease.

As you adjust to breast feeding, you may get sore, cracked nipples. We have some advice about sore nipples on page 59.

After about three months your breasts may change shape, or become a little smaller, especially if you are breast feeding. You can still have firm breasts if you follow the exercises on pages 104 and 117. And see Chapter 10 for breast maintenance.

Relaxin

The effects of relaxin on your ligaments puts joints at risk for up to five months after delivery. This can affect:

● lumbar spine (lower back)
● sacroiliac joints (hip bones)
● symphysis pubis (where the pubic bones join and where pain can be acute after childbirth)
● abdominal muscles
● pelvic floor (stress incontinence).

Do not overstretch as this can cause injury. Do all movements with control. You need to remember your posture, and you should try to adopt good posture when feeding and holding your baby.

Shaking

You may experience uncontrollable shaking in the early postpartum period. This shivering may be caused by nervousness and exhaustion related to childbirth, or may be a side effect of the extreme muscular exertion of delivery.

Your tummy

Your tummy will look five months pregnant for several weeks after childbirth, but it won't be firm. It is shrinking back every day but you will benefit greatly from doing the abdominal exercises in Chapter 7. If you still have a 'baby belly' after three months, don't worry, it will go (also see Chapter 7). If you were unable to avoid stretch marks, these may fade with the right type of skin nourishing (see page 81).

Pain during intercourse

Women who deliver vaginally often experience pain during intercourse, especially if they have had an episiotomy. Many doctors tell women it's fine to have sex after their six-week check up, but this may be too soon and cause discomfort, especially if you are breast feeding. Hormonal changes necessary for breast feeding can result in vaginal dryness, so a lubricant such as KY Jelly may help.

Endorphins

Huge amounts of endorphins, the 'feel good' hormone, are circulating round your body giving you an intense feeling of wellbeing. Many women assume that they will be exhausted straight after the birth, however, very often this is not the case.

Hair

Your hair, which may have got thicker during pregnancy will settle down after about three months, and you may shed hair quite dramatically as your hormone levels decrease. It will soon be replaced.

Breast feeding and weight loss

The quality of your milk is not always directly related to the quality of your diet, but the quantity of the milk usually is. The levels of protein, fat, and carbohydrate in your breast milk are not usually affected by the levels of these nutrients in your diet. However, the levels of some vitamins, for example vitamins A and B12, do depend on dietary intake. Your milk may be rich and good, but if you are not eating correctly, you may not have enough. To make good breast milk, and plenty of it, follow the dietary tips in Chapter 6, but increase your calorific intake by about 500 calories a day. If you have a lot of fat stores from your pregnancy (or before), you can take fewer calories, as the fat will be burned to produce milk, and you will lose some fat. If you are underweight, you will probably need more than 500 extra calories per day. No matter what your weight, you may find you need still more calories as the baby grows and demands still more milk.

Breast feeding may help you lose the excess weight from pregnancy, but it also makes you ravenously hungry, so you eat more anyway. By following our exercises and keeping good nutrition your weight will slowly drop away, leaving you with a lean firm body.

Emotional adjustment
A major factor in your ability and desire to get back into shape is your emotional adjustment, and much of that depends on your experience of labour and delivery.

Labour and delivery
Few mothers have the deliveries that they expect. We prepare as much as we can for labour and birth by attending

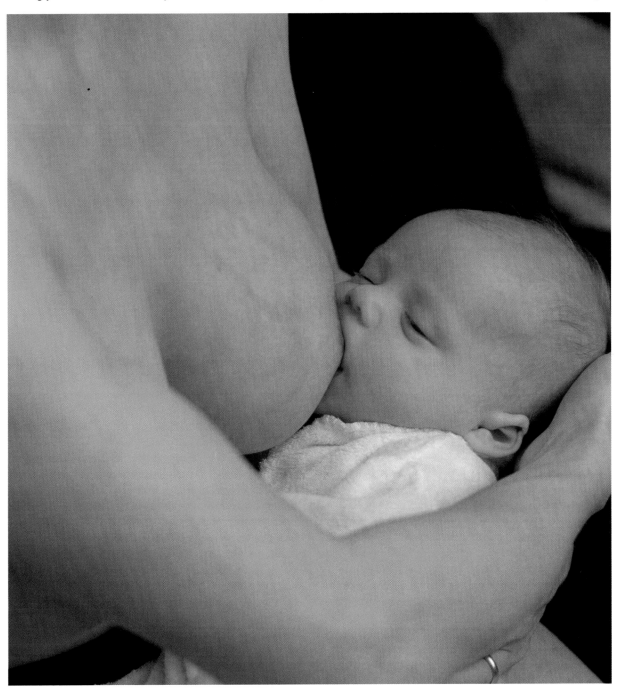

antenatal classes and trying birthing exercises and positions. Most of us hope that we can get through the pain of childbirth as naturally as possible, with little or no intervention, no medication, and feeling happy, complete, and peaceful afterwards.

If your labour was normal you will probably forget the pain as soon as your beautiful baby is put into your arms and you feel an overwhelming sense of protectiveness and responsibility. Hold your baby against your skin as soon as he is born so he can continue to hear your heartbeat. Mothers whose babies stay with them from birth onwards bond better and are more attentive to their babies' needs than those whose babies are taken away. If you have a caesarean section, or cannot hold your baby for some reason, state in your birth plan that you want your birth partner to hold your child first.

All aspects of the bonding process – your voice, smell, touch and caresses – are good for the baby. They are also good for you. The sooner you touch, hold, fondle and feed your baby, the sooner your bleeding will stop, the more strongly your uterus will contract down and the better your breasts will respond to the let down of colostrum and later milk.

Most of us will have a good experience of labour and birth, but those who do not, may feel inadequate if they don't live up to this ideal. Though once their baby is in their arms all is forgotten, a few women are left traumatised by their birth experiences.

It is hard to describe the pain of labour, and every woman will experience it differently. One thing that many women are unprepared for is the total loss of control. You are powerless to stop the pain, and have to rely on others to stop it for you. In an age when many women are used to having control of their lives, these women may find labour hardest because of this loss of power.

The relationship between a woman and her midwife is crucial to a happy childbirth experience. A midwife needs to be warm and sympathetic. If you have not had a positive experience of labour and birth, for whatever reason, it is important to talk to someone who can help you to make sense of what has happened. If these feelings are suppressed, anger may surface later.

Psychosocial changes

No one can prepare you for the changes a baby will make to your life. When you were pregnant, most of your thoughts were about your body, and the changes going on inside and around you. You wondered how all these changes would affect your relationships with your partner and friends. And you probably spent a lot of time towards the end of your pregnancy thinking about the birth and labour. How will it go? Will it hurt? Will I cope?

By now you will have realised that pregnancy and giving birth are the easy parts. Adjusting to a new baby and adapting your relationships with your partner, friends and family, will test your tolerance. Unless this extra stress is managed properly, you may become ill, physically or psychologically. If you are extremely stressed you may be unable to produce milk for your baby.

The postpartum period is the ideal time to adopt new life changes. We are ready to adopt new ideas that affect us psychologically and socially, and we will come to see that being relaxed and stress-free will help us to care for our new babies. As a result we may have a less demanding and more easy-going baby.

To successfully look after anybody else especially a baby we must first look after ourselves.

Stress
New mothers face many stresses: You may feel:
- extremely tired
- unprepared for motherhood
- anxious about your mothering skills
- anxious about childcare if you're going back to work
- unhappy about the state of your body
- unable to reorganise your life.

You will adjust more successfully to your new role if you know where all the potential stresses are coming from and can learn how to manage them effectively. Stress is our response to the situations thrown at us in daily life. To experience stress is a fact of life, and you will experience it with every change or adaptation in your life. The challenge is to prevent ourselves from becoming overstretched and experiencing detrimental effects that impinge on our health and ability to cope with everyday living.

Stress has two dimensions duration and intensity. Duration is more important for preventing illness and other adverse effects. We need to successfully manage stress so that it does not become a chronic problem. The postpartum period is demanding, but if you take breaks and adopt constructive ways of dealing with stress you can avoid any harmful results. Learning stress management techniques will have a positive effect on your relationship with your baby and any relationship that you have in life.

Stress might be positive such as having a baby or starting a successful business; or negative such as losing your job or marital difficulties. We can all choose how to deal with stressful situations. Our responses determine the amount of stress we will feel, not the situations themselves.

You can deal with stress constructively by:
● positive thinking
● organisation and time management
● rest and relaxation
● exercise and healthy nutrition
● use of humour
● meditation
● creating opportunities to cherish yourself.

Or destructively by:
● avoidance
● depression
● overeating
● using drugs
● loss of control.

Stress is not bad for you. Life would be quite boring if there were none. If you can manage stress successfully your life will have more excitement, motivation, and energy. Stress is only bad for you if you do not manage it effectively. Prolonged, unmanaged stress can lead to fatigue and exhaustion, depression, weight gain, and illness as our immune systems decrease their ability to function properly. Here we will look at some positive strategies for managing the stresses of the postpartum period. Chapter 10 will further explore other coping strategies to successfully manage the stresses of being a busy, modern mother.

Emotions

Having a baby is one of the greatest experiences in a woman's life. But many women go through a whole range of negative emotions sadness, anxiety, fear, anger, resentment after giving birth. Approximately seven out of ten women suffer from 'baby blues' where they feel tired and irritable for no reason. Baby blues may be due to a number of factors, for example:
● a dramatic drop in hormone levels after childbirth

● anxiety about baby and mothering skills
● fatigue and lack of sleep
● disillusionment over body condition.

Postnatal depression is a far more serious condition which requires medical attention.

The feelings you experience after the birth of your baby may be the most intense you have ever had. You may feel as though you have everything you ever wanted and yet you feel unhappy. Levels of oestrogen and progesterone plummet after childbirth, and these may trigger the blues in the same way that changing hormone levels can cause premenstrual tension. In some women the blues pass fleetingly on the third day when the milk comes in, or span a longer period while your hormones sort themselves out and you are beginning to make the emotional adjustments to having a new person in your life.

Your birth experience has a direct effect on how you feel afterwards. A good birth can make you feel strong, high, empowered and bond your relationships. But a traumatic birth can leave you feeling lost, in shock, empty and unable to cope.

Babies come in all different shapes, sizes, and temperaments. Some are calm others are very demanding. A woman with a demanding baby will need a lot more support than a woman with an easy-going baby. Though the mother with the good baby will still need support.

The stress of a new baby can show itself in different ways. Some women become more talkative, others become withdrawn. Some women overeat, others stop eating. I remember feeling shock and despondency at the thought that I might not have a good night's sleep for a long, long time.

Another problem, if you are feeling low, is believing everything that happens is out of your control, and you feel things are being thrust upon you from outside. When you are under pressure you can become blind to what is really happening around you.

All healthy relationships need compromise so that everyone can be happy. Your own needs are important, as are the baby's needs and those of your partner and family. Be open to the feelings that come to you day by day. Acknowledge and accept them. Talk about how you are feeling to people you trust, who care about you. Do not bottle up your emotions and do not listen to people who belittle your problems.

Positive Postpartum

Who can help

Talk to a sympathetic listener. It is good to keep in contact with at least one other new mum.

Talk to your health visitor. She has seen lots of women like you, and can tell you where to get help.

Homeopaths take emotional injury as seriously as physical injury so this would be a good time to go and see an accredited homeopath who will be able to treat the whole person.

Don't use food as a comforter. Keep a good balanced diet and do not overeat or binge on foods high in saturated fat. This will only make you put on weight, and make you feel even more unhappy.

Tackling fatigue

Fatigue and stress form a vicious circle. When you are tired, you are less able to manage stress successfully, which makes you more tired, and so on. Most women do not realise how long it can take to get back to normal. Labour and delivery are major physical events. While you are on a high after finally meeting your new baby, interrupted sleep will quickly take its toll on you and your partner. Constantly interrupted sleep is physically draining and psychologically upsetting for everybody. After childbirth, when your body is craving rest, the effects are greater. You may think you'll get the hang of motherhood in a couple of weeks, but many women feel more tired than ever two months after having their baby.

No other job is as physically draining and emotionally taxing. In most jobs the pressure is only on for eight hours a day, five days a week. A mother's job really is full time, with no lunch hours or tea breaks. If you are a first time mother you have the added worry of not being sure that you are doing the right thing. If this is your second or later child, you must juggle your time and emotions for each child. And you need energy to breast feed and carry your growing baby around. It all adds up to an exhausting routine. Newborn babies feed around the clock, and all have different feeding and sleeping patterns. On average they sleep for about 16 hours in 24. Unfortunately they cannot tell day from night, but as they grow they can take in more food, be more active between feeds and sleep for longer periods at night. By six months, most babies will have settled into a pattern.

Getting baby to sleep

The most important piece of advice is to sleep when your baby sleeps. You can help your baby establish a good sleep routine. Decide where and when you want him to sleep and stick with your decision. He should be ready for this between three and five months. If you are not firm, your baby will be confused, and you may find he is too tense and tired to sleep.

Sleep associations are important when teaching a baby to sleep by himself. From early on, think what you would like your baby to associate sleep with. Your bedtime routine, may include a bath, a clean nappy and changing into a sleepsuit. You may develop a ritual of saying good night to everyone, telling a story, giving a cuddle or singing a nursery rhyme. The crucial part is to make sure you leave the room while he is still awake.

Where your baby sleeps is also very important. Some mothers feel it is easier to have the baby in bed with them. Do what feels right for you and will give you maximum sleep. You need to:
● teach your baby to sleep by himself
● teach him to go back to sleep when he wakes at night.

How to prevent fatigue

Leave the housework. Stop worrying about the domestic chores, ask your partner or a friend to do the essentials.

Have the baby's cot right next to you or the baby in bed with you so you do not have to get up in the night.
Learn to relax. This will help if you find it hard to sleep during the day. We have some tips for relaxation in Chapter 10.

Express breast milk and let your partner share the care when the baby wakes at night.

Leave the nappy on. Only change the baby's nappy at night if you absolutely must. Modern disposable nappies are so well made they can be worn for the whole night without affecting the baby's skin.

Limit visitors. Restrict visits from friends and relatives unless they are willing to help out with the washing up or prepare a meal for you. When you are rested and in control, you will be able to entertain them.

Bring forward your own bedtime. Then the first night feed will not feel so awful if you have had a few hours' sleep.

Go with the flow. This is not the time to try to keep to a rigid routine. Relax and get to know your baby. If you're still in your dressing gown at suppertime, join the club. It will move back to lunchtime and eventually you will be dressed after breakfast.

If your baby cries when you're in the shower, it's OK. We're not saying leave your baby to cry, but that it's important that you take care of yourself. Having a shower and getting dressed will feel like a major achievement after days in your dressing gown. Look after your baby, then while he's content, or sleeping, look after yourself.

Don't try to be superwoman. When your baby is sleeping, you nap. If you are on your own, allow yourself an hour in the day when you will do whatever housework you can, then rest.

 Avoid stimulants like tea and coffee in the evening. If you are breast feeding, they will probably keep your baby awake too.

Eat well. Make sure that you are eating a good balanced diet, especially if you are breast feeding, and even if you are not. Make your treats part of your main meal your body will process them more efficiently, and you will probably enjoy them more.

Don't mistake fatigue for hunger. Your body is asking you to rest. Sit down, and if possible take a nap, not a biscuit or a piece of cake.

 Get out of the house as soon as you can even if it is just for a short walk. Low intensity aerobic exercise will relieve stress and tension, improve your mood, and will be energising. You and your baby will both benefit from being out in the fresh air, so take lots of walks.

 Try cocculus, china, kali phosphoricum, nitric acid, nux vomica, staphysagria or phosphoric acid.

Rest
This is the most important thing. If you are overtired you will not be able to think clearly. You must be aware of whether you are overdoing it or not.

Smile
This kids your subconscious into thinking you are happy and will make your body produce endorphins which will make you happy, which in turn will make you feel less tired.

Postnatal remedies

Note: For all homeopathic remedies, please see a registered homeopathic practitioner who will advise on dosages and duration of treatments.

Caesarean delivery
After a caesarean you can expect to feel tired. You not only have to deal with a newborn baby but you have to recover from an operation as well.

Take things at your own pace. Try to get up and walk around, but listen to what your body is telling you.

Try staphysagria, calendula or hypericum for severe pains in scars. If your scars are sore or lumpy and slow to heal try lachesis or silica.

Lavender oil will help you to relax and help your wound heal quicker. As soon as you are allowed to take a bath, add four drops of lavender to warm water. Relax in it for at least 10 minutes.

Sore perineum
Try arnica capsules or nux vomica.

If your perineum is sore, has torn or been stitched use these essential oils. As soon as the midwife agrees, add two drops of lavender and two drops of cypress oil to your bath or bidet, relax and try to soak for at least 10 minutes. You can use this up to three times a day and it is very soothing.

After pains
These are usually after second or subsequent deliveries. They can feel like period pains or more severe. The pain tends to be worse during breastfeeding. Try to breathe through the pain or find one of the comfortable positions you used in labour. Do not tense up this compounds the pain.
Try using arnica or magnesia phosphorica just before and during breast feeding.

Subinvolution
Sometimes the uterus does not contract down. This is called subinvolution. If your midwife thinks this applies to you, you may need to see your doctor.

Try cimicifuga, pulsatilla, sepia, caulophyllum, secale, carbo vegetabilis, carbonicum or staphisagria.

Positive Postpartum

Sweating

If you find yourself sweating more than usual as your body rids itself of excess fluid, try to avoid antiperspirants, as they tend to block the pores. Instead, use a crystallised mineral salt deodorant which is totally natural and hypoallergenic. These can be bought from most health food stores.

Engorged breasts

This is quite common and tends to happen a few days after birth when the milk comes in.

Try to rest more as engorged breasts can be a sign that you are overstressing yourself. Visualise your milk ducts flowing freely. The relaxing technique in Chapter 10 will help you to imagine your milk flowing out of your breasts. As the milk flows, help it along with some massage. Try massaging your breasts as the baby feeds, from the highest point down to the lowest to encourage the duct to clear. If you are engorged and also have a temperature, you have mastitis (blocked milk ducts) and you must seek help immediately. Use these remedies and also make sure your bra is not cutting in to you and causing a blocked duct. (Avoid wearing underwired bras.)

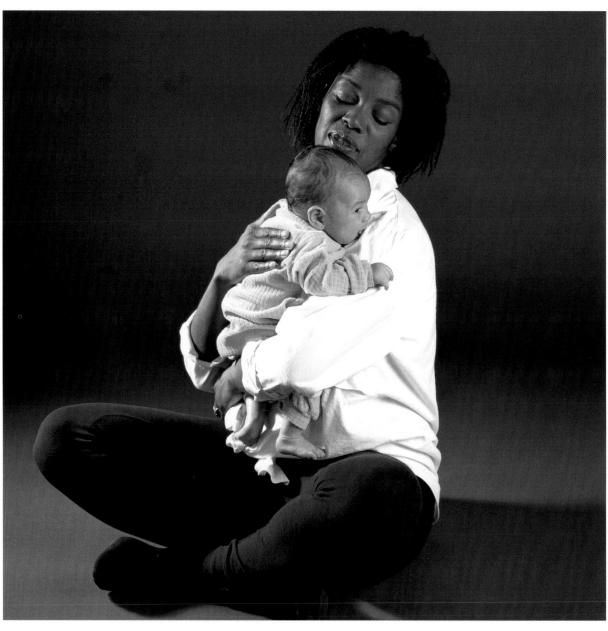

Keep cabbage leaves cold in the fridge and put them in your bra. This really helps as the cabbage draws out the excess heat. Change when the leaves become warm (unfortunately you will smell of boiled cabbage but for the relief it gives it is worth it).

 Homeopathic treatment is very successful at treating this. The two main remedies are belladonna and byronia. Stop taking arnica if you are taking it to recover from the shock of giving birth.

 To 300ml of either hot or cold water add two drops of lavender and two drops of geranium oil. Apply hot and cold compresses alternately to the sore breast.

Too little milk

 Sometimes our bodies need a little help with breastfeeding. Relax. If you are tense you will not let down milk as readily. Feed your baby often to encourage milk production, or try using a breast pump.

 Make sure you have eaten enough and that what you are eating is nutritious. Also make sure you are getting enough fluids: you will need about two pints more than you normally drink a day. Try drinking fennel tea as this promotes milk production.

Too little milk could be a sign that you are doing too much. Rest, and if possible get some help, so that all you have to do is feed yourself and your baby. Use the relaxation technique we suggest in Chapter 10.

 Try a short course of urtica urens.

Too much milk

If your milk is gushing out, your baby will choke and take in air which causes colic. This normally settles down within a few days.

 Place a sterile collecting shield against the non-feeding breast and collect the extra milk which you can then freeze and use later (you can buy these shields from supermarkets or chemists). Try expressing some milk before a feed if the milk is coming out too fast. During feeding sit your

baby upright so that he finds it easier to swallow. Let your baby feed just on one breast each feed (don't worry if your breasts become a bit lopsided they will even up once the milk supply settles down) After a feed apply a cold compress to slow down milk production.

Sore or cracked nipples

These can be very painful especially with your first child.

 Make sure the baby is 'latching on' properly, sucking on the whole of the nipple and the surrounding area, not just the tip. Your nipples can become sore if your baby is using them for comfort. Any more than about 10 minutes on each breast (with lots of swallowing and gulping sounds) tends to make them sore, so encourage the baby to suck on its thumb or your finger. Feed your baby as soon as she is hungry, very hungry babies latch on with great force. Let your nipples dry naturally before you put your bra back on.

Expose your nipples to the air as often as possible, especially after feeds. Do not wash your breasts too much, and never with soap. Another good treatment is to express a little milk and smooth onto the nipples, then allow the milk to dry naturally.

 Try phytolacca, borax, castor equi or sulphur remedies.

 Mix 20ml of aloe gel with three drops of rose oil and one drop of benzoin oil. Apply gel to the nipples after feeding, but remember to wipe it off before feeding (babies must not get essential oils in their mouths).

Weepiness

It is quite normal to feel a little weepy and lost for a few days after the birth.

 Try and get someone to help with baby and the housework. Have a bath if you can and wash your hair as well, as this seems to help.

 If you feel anxious try aconite or cimicifuga. If you feel weepy try pulsatilla or sepia.

 In your bath put up to five drops of any of these oils: clary-sage, bergamot, ylang-ylang, neroli or jasmin.

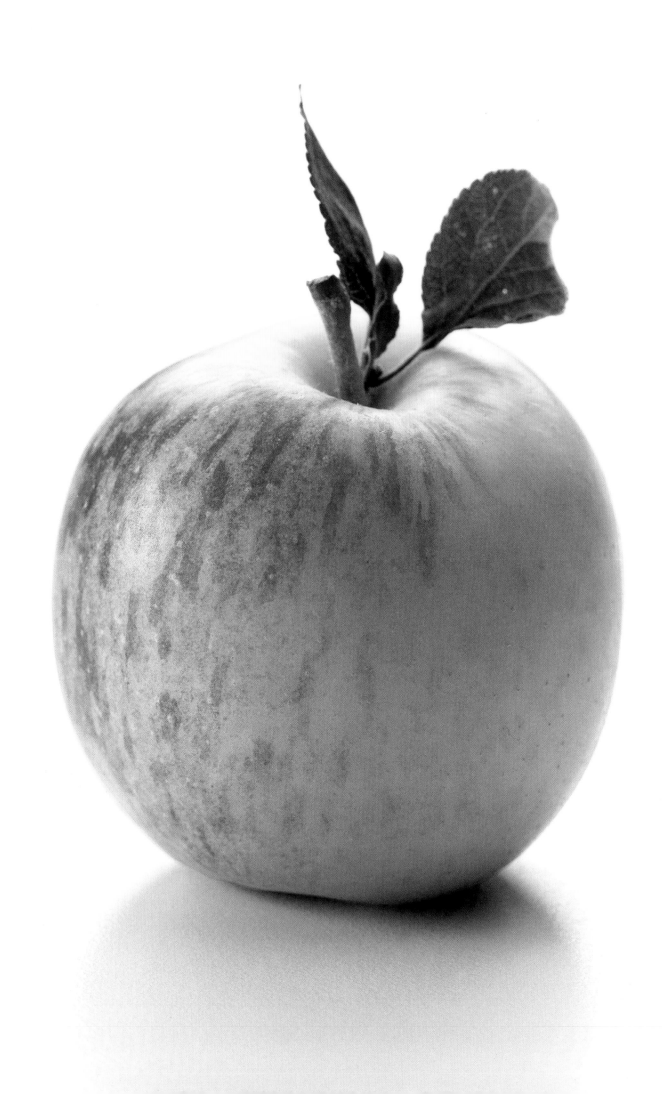

Nutrition

Have you heard of optimum nutrition? If you have, and you have adopted it into your lifestyle, you already have a well-balanced diet, rarely get colds or other infections, have high energy levels, firm skin and low body fat. If you haven't, read on.

Don't be daunted. The beauty of optimum nutrition is that it's so easy to incorporate into your way of life. It doesn't restrict your choice or deny you your favourite foods. And you will feel a change very soon after you start to follow the principles.

Optimum nutrition is eating the best nutrients to get the most out of your body and making it the healthiest that it can be. The balance of these nutrients has to be right for you. Too little is bad for you, and far too much is bad for you. Your needs are unique, and they depend upon other factors such as your genes, how active you are, your level of stress, and your environment. These nutrients are macronutrients – protein, carbohydrate, and fats; and micronutrients – vitamins and minerals.

Optimum nutrition is not about going on any sort of restrictive diet, and there is not one diet that applies to all. It is about adopting a completely new attitude to food. Already we are becoming more aware about avoiding foods with artificial additives, and eating less saturated fats and more fibre.

Optimum nutrition goes further. If you adopt it you will:
● eat whole foods
● eat more organic foods
● avoid trans fatty acids and hydrogenated fats
● eat less fried food
● make sure you are getting enough of the anti-oxidant vitamins A, C, and E and the minerals selenium and zinc to fight free radicals (see page 65) in the body and help prevent cancer and heart disease
● avoid drinking tap water
● become more aware of the potential dangers of genetically modified foods.

As a result you will be increase your wellbeing, and decrease your chances of suffering ill-health.

Good nutrition is the medicine of the future. There is proven scientific evidence that good nutrition, and eating certain foods can prevent and treat numerous diseases from the common cold to cancer. This is because some foods can direct biochemical events at the cellular level, where all health matters begin and end.

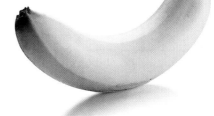

What is a balanced diet?

The modern diet consists of 40% fat, 12% protein, 48% carbohydrate (carbs) of which 20% is sugar.

Nutritionists generally accept that 60% carbs, 20% protein and 20% fat constitutes a balanced diet.

It takes a concerted effort in today's society to achieve a well balanced diet. The food industry is more concerned with profit than anything else. Many processed and manufactured foods are highly refined to make them last longer, but this process leaves them deficient in nutrients. We are being conditioned by the food industry to eat more and more sweet foods. There are vast amounts of sugar in children's foods, and with many mothers going out to work, we have to rely more and more on the availability of ready-made meals and sauces.

Proteins

Proteins are the body's chief building blocks. They are used to build muscles, bones, cartilage, skin and hair, and they circulate in the blood as hormones, enzymes and nerve chemicals. A good supply of protein is essential when you are pregnant or breast feeding, and during a strength training, fat burning programme.

Protein foods are beans, lentils, tofu (soya), some seed vegetables such as peas, corn and broccoli, meat, chicken, fish, nuts, cheese and eggs. Proteins are made up of combinations of 22 amino acids. Our bodies manufacture some of these amino acids, but the others we need to get from food. Examples of complete proteins with a full combination of essential amino acids needed for growth are eggs, soya, fish, chicken, and meat.

Some sources of protein are better than others. Meat can contain about 25% protein but up to 70% fat, much of it saturated. But meat contains some of the amino acids we need from our food. The best sources of protein are white meat and fish, and soya (tofu).

Carbohydrates

Carbohydrates are the body's chief source of fuel. They play a major role in influencing our appetites. Carbohydrates may be simple (sugars) or complex (starches and fibre).

Sugars

Simple carbohydrates (sugars) found in sweets and chocolate, are high in calories and provide instant energy. When you eat sugar, your blood sugar level rises dramatically, and your pancreas releases insulin into the bloodstream to stabilise this raised level.

Keeping your blood sugar balanced is one of the most important factors in maintaining energy levels and keeping your weight constant. When your blood sugar is low, you feel hungry. When it is high, for example, after a sugary snack, the release of insulin triggers a rapid drop in blood sugar, which makes you feel not only lethargic, but hungry again.

When there are high levels of sugar in the blood, the body converts the excess to glycogen in the short term, or fat our long term energy store. At the same time the high levels of insulin inhibits the breakdown of fat.

Blood sugar at the lower end of the range, leads to irritability, fatigue, poor concentration, and even depression. Diabetes results when the body cannot produce enough insulin to regulate blood sugar. This leads to a high blood sugar level and not enough glucose going to other organs.

Starches

Complex carbohydrates (starches) are the real energy foods. Grains, rice, potatoes and vegetables all contain large amounts of starch. Your body has to work harder to digest starches, even harder if they are unrefined, such as wholemeal bread, pasta and brown rice. This slows down your metabolism, provides you with long-lasting energy, keeps your blood sugar level constant, and keeps your appetite satisfied for longer.

Starches can be further divided into 'fast burning' and 'slow burning' starches, and high and low glycaemic indexes, which are also key to efficient use of food and fat reduction.

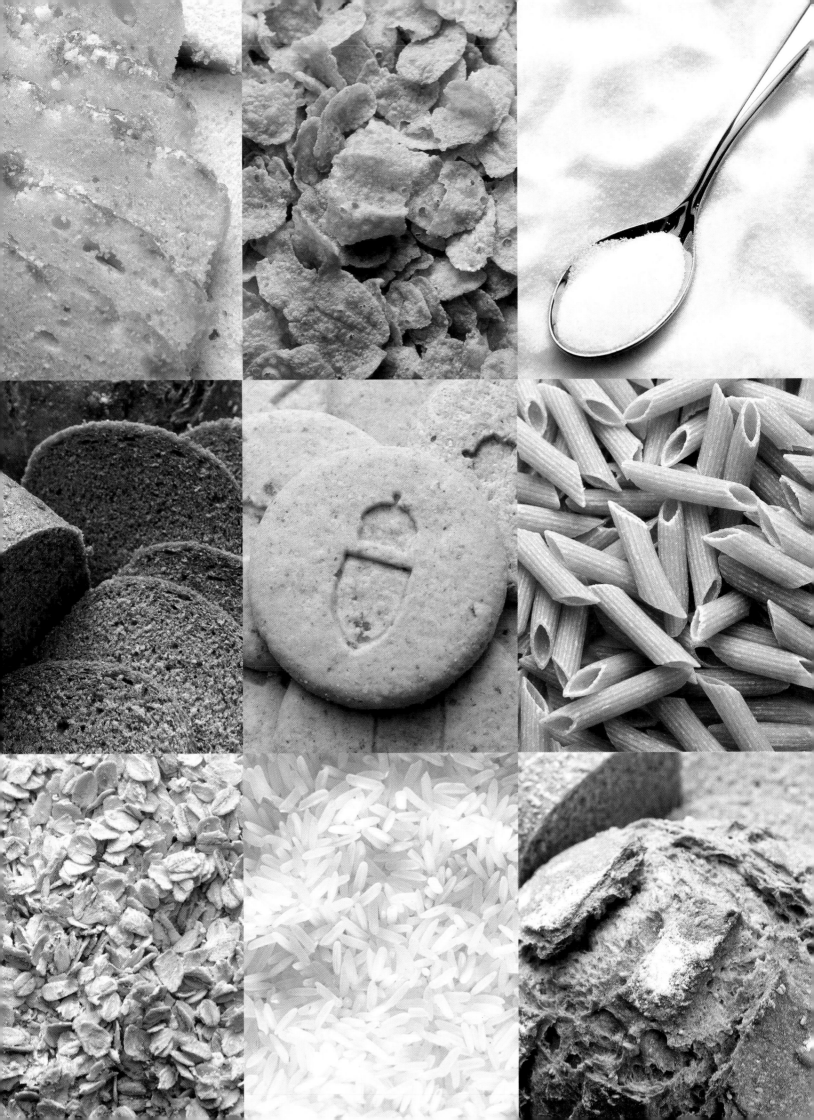

6

The glycaemic index

The glycaemic index of a food is the speed with which the carbohydrate in a food is broken down and turned into sugar to be released into the bloodstream. Sugary foods have a high glycaemic index, but not all starches have a low glycaemic index. Some fast burning starches are broken down into sugar quickly. Others take longer to be broken down.

Carbohydrate foods play a major role in influencing our appetites because they are broken down into glucose and enter the bloodstream. Falling and low blood sugar will trigger the appetite centres. Therefore, keeping blood sugar stable by eating predominantly low and medium glycaemic carbs, will give you greater energy and tame your appetite.

The glycaemic index also influences how much insulin is released into the bloodstream to stabilise the blood sugar level. For example, if you eat two slices of white bread, which has a high glycaemic index the sugar flow into your system will be rapid. The insulin response will be equally rapid, and again stimulating your appetite.

The glycaemic index of a food is also affected by the amount of protein or fat it contains. Protein and fat slow down the conversion of carbohydrate to sugar. Excess insulin also promotes the laying down of fat. You need to keep your blood sugar constant this will keep your energy level up and prevent fat from being deposited into body cells.

Try to eat some protein with each carbohydrate to slow down carbohydrate absorption, and prevent rapid rises in blood sugar.

Most foods with a high glycaemic index are over processed, calorie-dense and short on nutrients. Wholefoods usually have a low glycaemic index, are rich in nutrients and fibre, and have fewer calories for their weight.

The glycaemic index of some foods

Parsnips	97
White rice	87
Potato – baked	85
Potato – new	62
Cornflakes	84
Morning coffee biscuits	79
Watermelon	72
White bread	70
Wholemeal bread	69
Pineapple	66
Basmati rice	58
Oatmeal biscuits	55
Banana	55
Sweet potato	54
Pitta bread	57
Banana cake	47
All-bran	42
Porridge	42
Rye bread	41
Spaghetti	41
Apple	38
Pear	38
Cherries	22
Soya beans	18

Foods that have a low glycaemic index have a value below 55, intermediate glycaemic index foods have a value between 55 and 70, and high glycaemic index foods have a value over 70.

You should not necessarily avoid all high glycaemic index foods. We certainly do not recommend that you cut out rice from your diet. It is better to mix a high glycaemic food with a low glycaemic food or some protein or 'good' fats, so that the combination has an intermediate glycaemic index.

Fibre

There are two types of fibre – insoluble and soluble – and they have different roles in maintaining health and preventing disease.

Insoluble fibre in wheat bran, whole grains, and vegetables absorbs water in the digestive tract, increases stool bulk, speeds the movement of waste products through the digestive tract, and helps prevent colon cancer. In short, insoluble fibre is a natural laxative and will help prevent constipation during your pregnancy.

Soluble fibre is found in fruits, cooked dried beans and peas, oat bran, nuts and seeds. It has little effect on intestinal bulk, but it helps regulate blood sugar levels and lower blood cholesterol, thus helping prevent or to control diabetes and cardiovascular disease.

A fibre-rich diet is also filling and satisfying. It lets you eat more food for the same number of calories, and in the gut it helps to reduce the absorption of fat into the blood.

Left to right – good fats to bad fats.

Fats

When you're trying to lose fat and replace it with muscle, you may think of fat as the enemy, but it is not. We all need fat in our diets, but like carbohydrates, there are fats that will make you fatter, and fats that are an essential part of a healthy diet.

There are four kinds of fats:

● saturated
● polyunsaturated
● monounsaturated
● trans (hydrogenated) fats.

Saturated fats

Saturated fats such as beef fat, butter, lard, and palm oil are solid at room temperature. As well as making you fatter, eating too much saturated fat will also raise the level of cholesterol in the blood, which can clog the arteries and increase your risk of heart disease.

Polyunsaturated fats

Polyunsaturated fats such as sunflower oil and most vegetable oils are liquid at room temperature and only become firm if put in a freezer. Polyunsaturated fats help the body 'lose fat and protect it against heart disease. Your body cannot make these fats and they have to come from your diet. Your brain is 40% polyunsaturated fats, and breast milk is also high at 30%.

Certain polyunsaturated fats: Omega 3 (pumpkin and flax seed oils) and Omega 6 (sesame and sunflower oils) oils, are vital for the brain and nervous system. Omega 6 oils are converted in the body into DHA and EPA. These are found naturally in oily fish such as mackeral, salmon, tuna, and herring. Don't use polyunsaturated fats for cooking or they turn into trans fats.

Monounsaturated fats

Monounsaturated fats such as olive oil and peanut oil are liquid at room temperature and remain solid if chilled. Our bodies can synthesise these fats from other fats. These fats resist damage from free radicals and keep our blood vessels soft and pliable.

Trans fats

Trans fats, or hydrogenated fats, are polyunsaturated fats that are put through a process called hydrogenation that makes them hard. Your body treats trans fats as saturated fats, however they do not occur in nature and your body has not developed any mechanisms for making use of them except laying them down in your fat stores. Trans fats may also cause early ageing, skin troubles and other degenerative conditions.

Avoid them and anything that says 'hydrogenated vegetable oil' or 'partially hydrogenated vegetable oil' on the label. This list includes most margarines, most biscuits, cakes, and chocolate snack bars, and a lot of processed foods.

Antioxidants

If you cut an apple in half and leave it, the flesh of the apple will soon turn brown. This is oxidation. This is the reaction of oxygen in the atmosphere with the surface cells of the fruit. Although humans do not spoil the way that foods can, the cells of our bodies can be similarly damaged by the same chemical process of oxidation.

Oxidation produces free radicals, molecules that are missing an electron. They take electrons from other neighbouring cells to produce more free radicals. Free radicals are produced in all combustion processes such as frying,

smoking, barbecuing food, or burning toast. This cellular damage causes ageing, and can trigger other harmful chemical reactions such as cancers.

Oxidation can be kept in check by antioxidants, which are substances capable of disarming free radicals. Antioxidant vitamins include vitamin A and beta carotene, vitamin C, and vitamin E, as well as numerous phytochemicals (biologically active compounds in food not classed as nutrients) such as bioflavonoids found in citrus fruits.

How to change your eating habits for the better

This food plan is not set in stone. We aim to provide the guidelines, you can adapt it to suit you. If you enjoy a certain food, include it in the plan, and eat it at the right time. This plan is not about deprivation.

Remember:
- Eat the foods you like, and don't deprive yourself of the foods you love
- Don't rely on willpower alone, change the way you think about food, see it as the means to health and vitality
- Change your eating habits slowly, don't attempt it overnight
- Good nutrition is as much about what you don't eat as what you do eat

- Read all labels on the food that you buy and avoid anything that contains hydrogenated and trans fats
- Avoid eating too much fried food
- Try to eat plenty of low and intermediate glycaemic index carbohydrates in your daily diet
- Aim for three good meals daily, and two smaller snacks in between these meals
- Try to eat your last meal of the day as early in the evening as you can, and try not to eat anything afterwards (unless you are pregnant or breast feeding)
- Always eat breakfast, and try to make it a slow burning carbohydrate such as porridge oats
- Good nutrition goes hand in hand with exercise for total wellbeing.

A Good Day's Eating Plan

BREAKFAST
Porrridge oats with half a banana or some dried fruit to sweeten and skimmed milk
or Muesli with skimmed milk
or Boiled, poached, or fried egg (in a little olive oil) with a rasher of grilled, lean bacon and two slices of wholemeal bread.

MID-MORNING SNACK
Any one serving from the snacks table (see opposite).

LUNCH
Pasta with a low fat sauce containing tofu, tuna or lean mince and side salad
or Rice with vegetable and tofu stir fry or vegetables and grilled lean meat or fish
or if you're away from home,
Kebabs. Chicken kebabs are an excellent meal, high in protein, with carbohydrate from pitta bread and a good helping of salad. Avoid fatty Doner kebabs.
Sandwiches with a low fat filling. Pitta bread will satisfy you longer than ordinary bread because of its mid-glycaemic index value.

MID-AFTERNOON SNACK
Any single serving from the snacks table.

DINNER
Similar to lunch with a slightly higher protein content and slightly lower carbohydrate content.

If you are pregnant or breast feeding, you may need a snack later in the evening after dinner, choose a low-mid glycaemic index snack from the snacks table.

Carbohydrates
Aim for 5-6 servings daily. Each serving contains between 20 and 25 grams of complex carbohydrate. Choose from the following:
- 2 slices of bread
- 120g (half a cup) cooked rice (basmati has a lower glycaemic index than white long grain)
- 130g pasta
- 1 sweet potato
- 2 fist sized potatoes
- a large bowl of porridge.

Proteins
Aim for 4 servings daily. Each serving contains between 18 and 25 grams of protein. Choose from the following:
- 3 glasses of skimmed or semi-skimmed milk
- 65g /(three quarter) tub of low-fat cottage cheese
- 125g of low fat yoghurt
- 55g of cheese
- 2 large whole eggs plus 2 egg whites
- 100g fish
- 75g chicken or turkey (no skin)
- 80g of lean beef, lamb, pork or dark meat chicken
- 50g tofu
- 1 serving of a complete protein supplement, such as whey protein powder
- 250g of beans or pulses e.g. lentils
- 100g hummus (low fat variety)
- 1 tablespoon of peanut butter.

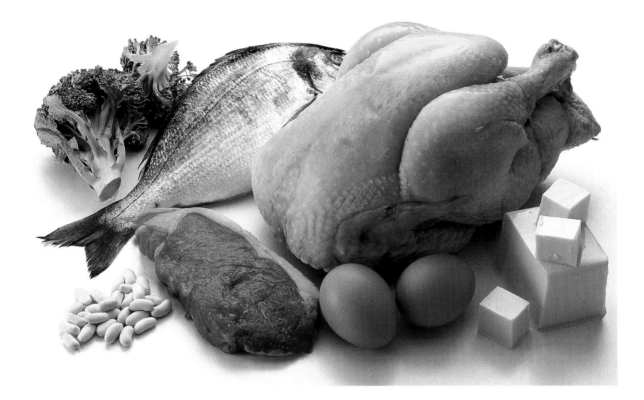

Snacks

How to reduce your intake of sugar

Avoid sugary and fat loaded chocolate bars, try instead any of these:

- a handful of dried fruit and nuts
- a wholemeal bun and a piece of fruit
- 3 organic oatmeal biscuits
- biscuits or cookies made with oats, soyflour, sesame or sunflower seeds, or calcium-rich carob
- bran muffin and fruit
- 2 ryvita with cottage cheese or peanut butter

Good fats

(4 full or 8 half-servings)

Half servings

- 30g of cheese
- 1½ tablespoons single cream
- 175ml/ 6 fl oz whole milk
- 225ml/ 8 fl oz semi-skimmed milk
- 1 egg or egg yolk
- half a small avocado
- 75g tofu

Full servings

- 1 tablespoon of polyunsaturated cold pressed vegetable oil, e.g. flaxseed, sunflower, safflower, soya or canola oil
- 1 tablespoon olive oil
- a starflower oil supplement
- 1 tablespoon peanut butter
- 1 tablespoon of butter
- 125g of canned salmon, mackerel, sardines or herrings.

How to reduce your intake of bad fats

- Use fats and oils sparingly
- Read the nutrition facts label on the packaging avoid anything that says 'hydrogenated' or 'partly hydrogenated'
- Eat plenty of grain products, vegetables, and fruit; the fibre helps to reduce the absorption of fat into the blood
- Choose low fat milk products, lean meats, fish, poultry, beans, and peas to get essential nutrients without increasing your intake of calories and saturated fats.

Antioxidants

- Fruit such as oranges, grapefruit, red and black grapes, strawberries (vitamin C, poly phenols and flavanoids)
- Vegetables such as carrots, sweet potatoes, broccoli, cabbage, and fruit such as peaches and apricots (beta carotene vitamin A)
- Sesame seeds (vitamin E).

Fibre

Aim for 5 servings daily. Choose from the following:

- 2 slices of wholemeal bread
- use wholewheat pasta instead of white pasta
- 1 piece of fruit
- porridge and oatbran cereal
- 50g vegetables or large bowl of salad
- cooked dried beans or peas.

Healthy eating in pregnancy

What you eat before and during your pregnancy is the most important determinant of your health and that of your unborn child. Poor maternal nutrition can have serious effects on the growing baby. From conception to birth and the months following birth, if you breast feed, your baby is totally dependent on you. You provide all the essential nutritional building blocks your baby needs for the growth and development of every cell, tissue, organ, and system in his body.

Pregnancy, when your body is in its most natural state, is the ideal time to adopt a pattern of good, healthy nutrition and keep to it. Your skin, your hair, your body, and your brain are all physically made up of what you eat. And so is your baby's. A child who is born strong and healthy will have fewer illnesses throughout life than a child who is born with a low birth weight.

This responsibility is great but not daunting, you just need to use a little nutritional common sense. Quality is the key when choosing nutritious foods. Focus on minimally processed, wholesome foods.

The good news is that eating a healthy diet – an optimum nutrition diet – is even easier when you are pregnant. If you are suffering from nausea, healthy eating can help the condition. If you let your body take over, and only eat what your body draws you to, you will naturally eat foods that are nutritious for yourself and your baby. You will have the odd craving for a chocolate eclair, but as long as you eat such treats in moderation, and at the right time, they can fit into your optimum nutrition plan.

Weight gain

It doesn't take a dietary genius to realise that the more you eat, especially the 'empty' calories of high sugar foods, the more weight you will put on. And research has shown that excess weight gain during pregnancy makes you less likely to go back to your pre-pregnancy size.

Although we have no set figures in this country, we accept the American guidelines of 25-35lbs for healthy weight gain during pregnancy. If you are of average weight you need only about 300 calories more than normal to maintain your pregnancy weight, though this also depends on your level of activity. Pregnancy is not the time to try and lose weight. Eating fewer calories than your body needs is potentially dangerous and can affect the development of your baby.

On the other hand, consuming too many calories can compound many pregnancy problems and means extra weight to burn off after the baby is born. The amount of fat cells your baby has is determined while your baby is inside you and in the first year of life, so you must be careful not to eat a diet that is too high in fat. The extra calories should be made up of nutrient rich foods.

Before conception

Ideally, you should begin preparing for pregnancy months before conception, especially if your diet has been less than perfect up to now. If you're nutritionally prepared, you will be ready for the first few weeks of your baby's life, when cell changes and growth are so rapid that all her vital organs are formed.

Eating well before pregnancy helps prepare you for the nutritionally intense nine-month period of making a baby. Of the 50 essential nutrients needed for the growth and healthy development of your baby, two are particularly important before you conceive:

● folic acid
● iron.

Folic acid

Consuming a folic acid rich diet or taking a multivitamin and mineral supplement with folic acid at least six weeks before conception, and for the first few months of pregnancy, significantly reduces your baby's risk of developing neural tube defects such as spina bifida. Folic acid is essential even if there's no history of birth defects in your family.

Because folic acid goes to work in the first few weeks of pregnancy, it's a good idea for all women of childbearing age to make sure that they consume one or two folic acid rich foods every day, or take a multivitamin supplement that contains 400 milligrams of folic acid.

Iron

Iron is the oxygen carrier in the body. If you have too little iron your tissues are literally starved of oxygen, leaving you feeling tired, mentally confused, and susceptible to colds and infections. Iron deficiency also reduces your ability to tolerate blood loss during labour.

During pregnancy, your developing fetus and your increasing blood supply will take a toll on your iron reserves. If you're low in iron, or are anaemic due to iron deficiency, your doctor may recommend some iron supplements, or you can buy herbal-based iron supplements that are easily absorbed, at your local health food store. You can yourself increase your consumption of iron rich foods to make sure that you get your 15mg of iron daily.

From the moment of conception, your baby needs all of the 13 essential vitamins including vitamins A, E, D, K, C, and the B vitamins, such as B6, B12, and folic acid for growth and development.

Folic acid
(RDA in pregnancy 400mcg)
Aim for two servings daily. Choose from the following:
- 4 asparagus spears
- half an avocado
- 1 serving cooked dried beans and peas
- a serving of dark green leafy vegetables such as spinach, greens, romaine lettuce, broccoli
- 150ml orange juice
- 30g sunflower seeds
- 2 tablespoons wheat germ.
- 2 slices of wholemeal, fortified bread.

Iron
(RDA in pregnancy 15mg)
Small amounts of iron are found in most fruits, vegetables, grains and meat, but try to have some of the following higher iron content foods daily, along with your supplement (if you take one).

- lean duck or chicken
- cooked oysters
- sardines
- dark green leafy vegetables
- iron fortified cereals
- tofu
- pumpkins
- carob or carob flour
- blackstrap molasses
- dried fruit.

Vitamins

The fat-soluble vitamins

Vitamin A is essential for the development and maintenance of your baby's immune system, vision, bones, skin and the lining of the internal organs. However, large doses of this vitamin·can be harmful to your developing baby, so don't take supplements above 2,000 iu per day.

Beta carotene supplies vitamin A.

Vitamin D helps form a baby's bones and prevents rickets, a disorder characterised by bone deformities. Vitamin D can be toxic if taken in large amounts.

Vitamin E is an antioxidant that protects the body from damage and helps form normal blood cells, muscle cells, and other tissues.

Vitamin K aids in blood clotting and may promote bone formation.

The water soluble vitamins

Vitamin C Your baby needs Vitamin C for proper growth and the development of strong teeth and bones. It is essential to the formation and maintenance of collagen, a protein that

Nutrition

6

Box 2. The best food sources of essential vitamins.

Vitamin	Food sources
Vitamin A	liver, eggs
Beta carotene	dark green or orange vegetables, cantaloupe, peaches, apricots
Vitamin D	fortified milk, fatty fish, egg yolks
Vitamin E	wheat germ, safflower oil, spinach
Vitamin K	dark green leafy vegetables
Vitamin B1	whole grains, wheat germ, brewer's yeast, peanuts, green peas, dark green leafy vegetables
Vitamin B2	milk, avocados, dark green leafy vegetables, salmon, asparagus
Niacin	chicken, fish, peanut butter, green peas, wheat germ, brewer's yeast
Vitamin B6	chicken, fish, avocados, potatoes, bananas
Folic acid	dark green leafy vegetables, strawberries, orange juice, wheat germ
Vitamin B12	meat, chicken, fish, eggs, milk
Biotin	oatmeal, soya beans, peanut butter, fish, milk, brown rice
Pantothenic acid	chicken, fish, eggs, milk, peanut butter, bananas, oranges, brown rice, wheat germ
Vitamin C	citrus fruits, brussels sprouts, strawberries, tomatoes, potatoes, dark green leafy vegetables

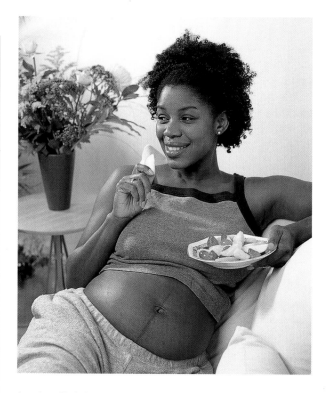

bonds cells in bones, teeth, tendons, skin, the cornea of the eye, and blood-vessel walls. Vitamin C improves the absorption of iron in the body and counteracts some of the inhibitors of iron absorption, such as phytates in whole grains and tannins in tea and coffee. It also plays a role in hormone activity. Your body cannot store vitamin C so it must be taken in every day.

B vitamins, especially vitamins B1, B2, niacin and biotin, work as a team in energy production, muscle and nerve development, the development of essential fats, and the general growth of your baby. Vitamin B6 is essential to the development of your baby's nervous system and for protein metabolism. Vitamin B12 is needed for red blood cell formation.

Many of the B vitamins also promote the mother's circulation so that nutrients can get to the baby more efficiently. Some B vitamins, such as pantothenic acid and vitamin B6, are important in the production of hormones and in the formation of the pigment in haemoglobin (the protein in red blood cells). Box 2 shows the best sources of essential vitamins.

Box 3. The best food sources of minerals.

Mineral	Food sources
Calcium	milk products, sardines, canned salmon with bones, tofu (firm), dark green leafy vegetables, dried beans and peas
Chromium	whole grains, wheat germ, orange juice
Copper	chicken, fish, meats, avocados, potatoes, soybeans, dark green leafy vegetables
Iodine	milk, eggs, seafood, some breads, Iodised salt
Iron	lean meats, dried apricots, dark green leafy vegetables, raisins, dried beans and peas, potatoes with skin
Magnesium	low fat milk, peanuts, bananas, wheat germ, dark green leafy vegetables, oyster
Manganese	raisins, spinach, carrots, broccoli, oranges, green peas
Molybdenum	lean meats, whole grains, dried beans and peas, dark-green leafy vegetables
Phosphorus	meats, chicken, fish, milk, yogurt, eggs, grains, beans, nuts
Potassium	fruits, vegetables, fish, peanuts, potatoes
Selenium	whole grains, seafood, lean meats and low-fat milk products
Zinc	lean meats, turkey, dried beans and peas, wheat germ

Minerals

Iron has been mentioned on page 69.

Calcium During the first six months of pregnancy, a mother's calcium-rich diet must provide her baby with up to 300 mg of calcium daily to build his skeletons and teeth. Calcium is also vital for muscle, heart, and nerve development, blood clotting and enzyme activity. To replenish this calcium, you need to consume at least 1,200 mg of calcium per day the equivalent of four glasses of low-fat milk.

Calcium is not only very important for strong teeth and bones - if you do not take in enough calcium for your baby's growth, your body will give its own calcium, taken from your bones which will set you up for osteoporosis in later life.

Other essential minerals are:

Magnesium for energy, muscles, and nerves

Chromium for the normal regulation of blood sugar

Copper for the development and maintenance of your baby's heart, arteries and blood vessels

Iodine, a component of the hormone thyroxine, which regulates the metabolism for you and your baby

Selenium, an antioxidant mineral that protects red blood cells and cell membranes from damage and is important in maintaining a strong immune system. Selenium can be toxic if taken in high doses. So eat selenium-rich foods but limit selenium supplements to below 100 mcg per day

Zinc facilitates conception, so it is essential from the very start of pregnancy. During pregnancy, zinc helps to maintain normal tissue growth.

Good fats

Polyunsaturated fats

One of the latest developments in dietary advice in pregnancy is the increasing emphasis on the value of polyunsaturated fats. These 'good' fats are needed to promote brain, eye and body growth in the baby. As they are not made in the body they are essential to the diet.

DHA

Docosahexaenoic acid (DHA) is a member of the Omega 3 family. Its benefits during pregnancy and while breast feeding are becoming more widely known.

About 600 million years ago DHA was responsible for the evolution of human sight, the nervous system, and sensitivity to light. Every movement we make, our speech, thoughts and vision are influenced by the DHA present in the brain. It is vital for the proper development of a baby's brain, nervous system, and retina. Research has shown that taking extra DHA can improve your chances of giving birth to a larger child and reduces the risk of prematurity.

The richest source of DHA is oily fish, such as herring, mackerel, salmon, and tuna. Fresh tuna oil is the richest natural source of DHA. Breast milk contains DHA. DHA is vital in the third trimester when the baby's brain has rapid growth spurts. 70% of the baby's calories are used for growth and development of the brain at this stage.

One source of DHA is Milkarra Oil capsules, (available from The Pregnancy Shop) which contain tuna fish oil and evening primrose oil.

Fibre

Most women experience some digestive tract problems during their pregnancies. Most of these problems, from constipation to haemorrhoids, can be avoided or minimised if you add a little fibre to your daily diet (see page 67).

Salt

In the past, pregnant women were warned to limit their salt intake to manage their weight gain and prevent swelling and high blood pressure. Now we know that pregnant women need some salt in their diets to maintain their increasing blood volume, which increases by up to 40%. Your cells also hold more water during pregnancy. A little bit of swelling is normal starting in the second trimester, and especially in the final few weeks.

This mild fluid retention is unrelated to salt intake, and shouldn't be treated by restricting salt or taking diuretic medications (water tablets) without your doctor's approval.

Water

Water is important in all biological processes. Without it, the body's functioning stops.

You should try to drink at least eight glasses of filtered or bottled water per day. If you drink a glass when you wake up, one before each meal, and one at bedtime, you're almost there.

Too many caffeinated beverages and fizzy drinks can have a diuretic effect: they increase the flow of urine and make you dehydrated. Juices can be a good addition to your diet as long as they are not artificially sweetened. They can increase your caloric intake.

Exercise causes massive water loss through sweat, so if you are exercising, you should increase your water intake by one or two glasses an hour before exercise, and another one or two afterwards.

Foods to avoid when you are pregnant

Listeria infection is very rare, but can lead to miscarriage, stillbirth, or severe illness in the new-born. The following foods should be avoided because of the risk of listeria:

Pate, unpasteurised goat's, cow's, or sheep's milk or cheese, blue veined cheeses (Stilton, Danish blue), soft cheeses, undercooked ready meals, salads chopped for more than 24 hours.

To avoid **salmonella** poisoning, avoid raw or undercooked eggs, home-made mayonnaise, shellfish, and desserts such as ice cream, tiramisu, and chocolate mousse.

Toxoplasmosis is an infection caused by a parasite found in meat, cat faeces, and soil. The infection can be harmful to unborn babies so good hygiene is essential especially when handling raw meat, changing cat litter or gardening. Wear gloves or ask someone else to do it.

Drugs

While you are pregnant, you should avoid alcohol, tobacco and medications (unless prescribed by your doctor). Alcohol can cause permanent physical and mental birth defects. Since no safe limit has been established for alcohol consumption, abstinence is your best bet for safety.

Drinking alcohol and smoking are harmful to unborn babies, and doing both is compounding the risk. New research has confirmed that development of babies in the womb is disrupted when they are exposed to alcohol and tobacco. Researchers tested the unborn babies at 25 weeks using a startle reaction to noise. Among mothers-to-be who smoked and drank, two-thirds of the babies failed to react, compared with less than a third of mothers who neither smoked nor drank. It is best to avoid both tobacco and alcohol during pregnancy and after childbirth, especially if breast feeding.

Treats

If you want to eat a chocolate bar or a packet of crisps, do, but after you have eaten something nutritious. Do not substitute junk food for your normal diet. Eat something good first then have your treat. If you do it the other way round, you fill up on low nutrient, high fat foods and then do not want to eat the good foods.

Organic foods

Unfortunately most of the world's foods are grown with the use of pesticides and herbicides, artificial fertilisers and other chemicals and drugs. Some toxic substances for example the pesticide DDT have now been banned.

There are legal limits to the amount of dangerous chemicals allowed in our foods, but new chemicals are being continually introduced, and regulations cannot keep up. During pregnancy and during their first year of life babies are particularly vulnerable because they are growing very rapidly and so take in large amounts of food in relation to the small size of their bodies. Their livers are not yet ready to deal with toxic substances.

The best way to avoid these chemicals is to eat organic foods, which are produced without the use of artificial chemicals. Organic fruit and vegetables are grown in orchards and fields that have not been sprayed or fertilised with artificial chemicals. Organic meat and dairy produce come from animals that have grazed on grass grown with natural fertilisers, and have eaten fodder free from drugs and other chemicals.

It is difficult, and expensive, to eat totally organic, but a good rule is that the closer to the ground the product is, the more contaminated it is likely to be. For example, vegetables grown under the ground, like carrots or potatoes, are more likely to have absorbed artificial pesticides and fertilisers. The same goes for low grown soft fruits like strawberries. If possible at least try to buy these products organically.

When choosing whether or not to buy organic, a good general rule is that if you or your children eat a lot of a certain food, buy organic.

Apples, pears, and peaches

Conventionally grown samples often contain high pesticide levels. Organic apples also have higher levels of vitamin C and potassium.

Strawberries, raspberries, and blackberries

Many conventionally grown strawberries and other soft skinned fruits are treated with methyl bromide a toxic soil fumigant which is dangerous to animals and birds and also depletes the ozone layer.

Carrots

Organic carrots have a much higher amount of dry matter and taste better.

Celery

Tests have shown conventionally grown celery sticks to contain more than the 'acute reference dose' the amount of pesticide which can be consumed in a single portion without causing adverse reactions.

Potatoes

Standard crops are fertilised with nitrates and supply a third of the nitrate in the diet. Boiling reduces the concentration of nitrates, frying does not. Eating organic potatoes reduces the intake of nitrates, which can be converted to potentially carcinogenic substances in the stomach.

Lettuce

In recent years, three growers have been prosecuted for using illegal fungicide on conventionally produced lettuces.

Tomatoes

Despite a falling level of pesticide use, residue levels in tomatoes are still highly unpredictable.

Spinach

Eating only 130g (one generous serving) of spinach a day would exceed the recommended levels of nitrate. Organic spinach has lower levels

Tofu

Always buy organic to avoid consuming genetically modified soy.

Beef

Organic beef is not better nutritionally, but it comes with a guarantee that the meat is BSE-free.

Liver

Always buy organic, the liver filters out all the toxins from the body

Chicken and poultry

Conventional poultry production can still involve routine dosing with low level drugs, contributing to the problem of antibiotic resistance. Though it's not organic, free range poultry is reared along organic lines.

Milk and yoghurt

Conventionally produced milk can sometimes contain lindane, an organochlorine insecticide that affects hormone activity and has been linked to breast cancer. There was an unexpected rise in 1995, but recent tests have not found levels above the Maximum Residue Level (MRL). We recommend organic milk and yoghurt for pregnant women and children.

Eggs

Free range eggs, though not nutritionally better, are kinder to the birds.

Wine

It's estimated that the production of cheap (under £5 per bottle) mass market wines accounts for nearly half the pesticides applied to arable land.

Apple juice

If you drink a lot, go for organic because of the pesticide residues sometimes found in apples.

Grains

Wholemeal bread, wholewheat pasta and brown rice are far more likely than refined cereals to contain pesticide residues because they retain the outer layers of the grain.

Organic peanut butter may be healthier and tends to have less or no added salt.

Chocolate

Organic versions are healthier and better for teeth because they are often made with more cocoa solids and less sugar. Conventional cocoa production uses large amounts of insecticides that inflict environmental damage.

Healthy eating after childbirth

You don't need any special foods after childbirth, but you should continue to eat healthily, and take a multivitamin to make sure that you are getting enough vitamins and minerals during a potentially stressful time when you may not be paying enough attention to your diet. The weight loss will come with the fat burned from increased physical activity and cutting down on sugary foods.

If you are breast feeding, your body burns more calories every day to produce the milk. Once it was believed that this calorie expenditure helped the mother to lose baby fat, but tests have shown that you consume more calories while breast feeding, so negating this effect.

Breast feeding and exercise will increase your metabolism, but you need to watch what you eat not only to prevent weight gain, but also to provide your baby with the best nourishment possible. Try to eat three or more servings of calcium rich foods such as broccoli, cauliflower, and dairy foods. Quality of milk is more important than quantity when you are breast feeding.

You also need to make sure that you are well hydrated when you are breast feeding. You need the extra fluid for your milk. When you exercise and your body starts to shed its baby fat, you need to drink plenty of water. The fat has to go into the bloodstream before it is excreted out of your body, so you need lots of water to flush your organs and to prevent your system becoming too acidic from the broken down fat. The minimum you should be drinking is 6 to 8 glasses of water a day.

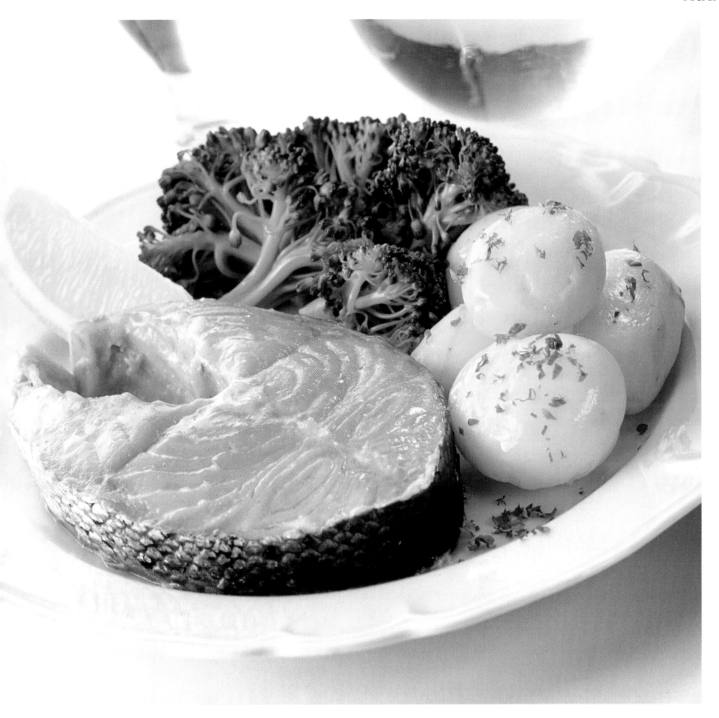

The habit of a lifetime

When you've given birth and you are looking at all those clothes that used to fit you, avoid the temptation of going on a temporary restrictive diet to get your figure back. Our programme is about making permanent changes in your life. As you see the progress you make when you eat more healthily and take exercise, you'll find it easier to make this the habit of a lifetime.

Further reading

The Optimum Nutrition Bible. Patrick Holford.
The G.I. Factor. Dr Anthony Leeds, Professor Jennie Brand-Miller, Kaye Foster Powell & Dr Stephen Colagiuri

7

The Waist

Your abdomen is a part of your anatomy that is greatly affected by pregnancy. If there is one single burning question that new mothers ask about fitness, it is: 'Will I ever get my figure back?' A leading women's magazine recently asked 6,000 women how they felt about their bodies. The tummy came top of the least-liked list: nearly half the women named their tummies as the least favourite part of their anatomy.

Looking at your tummy during the later stages of pregnancy and immediately after childbirth, you may fear you'll never have a waistline again. It is truly a wonder of nature to see a fully pregnant tummy spring back to a small waist and flat tummy after childbirth.

Following delivery, the abdominal wall is very loose and stretched. A large portion of the postpartum abdomen distension is fat, poor muscle tone, and stretched surface skin. For a lucky few, most of this takes care of itself within two or three months after giving birth.

Some of us are not so lucky. Without a concentrated effort to practise abdominal exercises designed to tighten and strengthen our abdominal muscles ('abs'), we are left with a protruding pouch in the lower abdomen, often long after we have had our babies. And some are left with a surplus of loose skin there.

This chapter is all about getting your waist back, and regaining or gaining for the first time a flat tummy after your baby is born. It rarely happens naturally, and

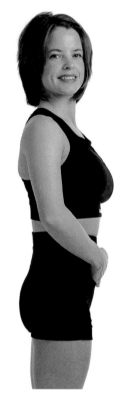

most of us need to work at it. By concentrating on the waist while it is expanding during pregnancy, we show you how your waist can spring back into shape, and often end up smaller than it was before you were pregnant by focussing on:

● Special exercises for the abdominal muscles
● Good posture
● Skin condition
● Good nutrition

Don't despair if your baby is one, 10 or even 21 years old and you still have a baby belly, you can get rid of it naturally. I got rid of mine, and I'll show you how.

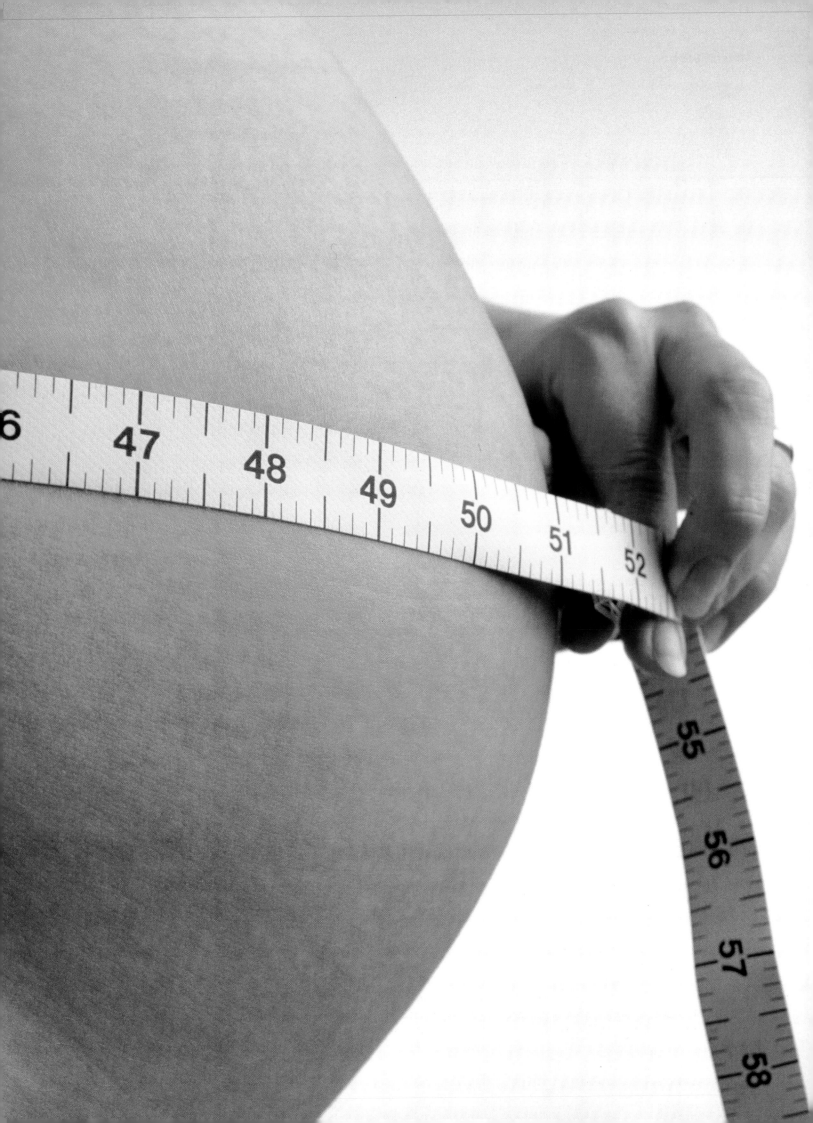

7

The Abdominal Muscles

The abdominal muscles ('abs') consist of several muscle groups. The **rectus abdominus** is one long, continuous muscle, made up of two halves, which extends from your pubic bone to your ribs. This muscle is stretched during pregnancy to accommodate the growing baby, and separates mid line.
See figure 1.

Abdominal support is assisted by a corset of muscles which collectively form the waist area. These include the **internal and external obliques**, which help you to bend and rotate.
See figure 2.

The **transversus abdominus** is your deepest abdominal muscle, and runs from just inside your obliques, and right round your back.
See figure 3.

Last, but not least, your **pelvic floor** muscles. This hammock of muscle runs under your body from your pubic bone to your tailbone. It supports the growing weight of the baby, and all your internal pelvic organs the bowel, bladder and womb. It stretches to its maximum during delivery. Greater strength and control of your pelvic floor muscle can assist the abdominals, and correctly re-strengthening this muscle after childbirth helps to regain abdominal control.

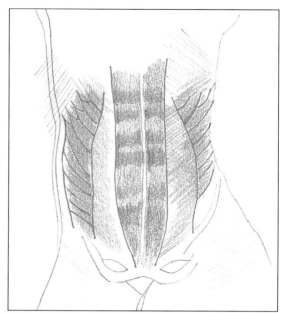

figure 1.

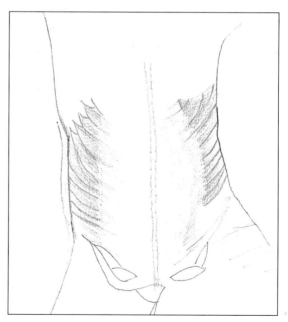

figure 2.

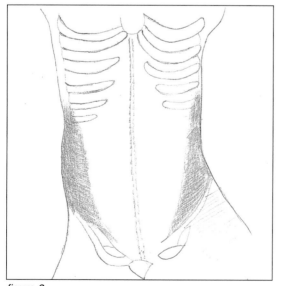

figure 3.

Let gravity help

Because humans walk in an upright position, your centre of gravity when you are pregnant is constantly shifting as your baby grows. This stresses the back and joints. But if you are on your hands and knees, all these stresses are reduced. The growing weight of your baby is now used along with the pull of gravity as a weight for strengthening rather than weakening.

Exercises practised on all fours become optimal during pregnancy, and just after delivery. They increase circulation, which can in turn help prevent or relieve conditions such as haemorrhoids, varicose veins, cramp and indigestion. Isometric (using minimum movement and maximum tension or contraction) abdominal strengthening exercises in this position are safe and effective.

Exercises to avoid

If you exercise in an upright, weight bearing position using gravity as a resistance you can weaken your abdominals and stress your pregnant body. For this reason it is recommended that you avoid the following activities

● step or bench aerobics
● high impact aerobics
● jogging (unless familiar and comfortable with it).

Also, in the second and third trimester avoid:
any abdominal exercise that involves lying on your
back or any leg exercises that involve you resting on
your hands and knees with one leg in the air.

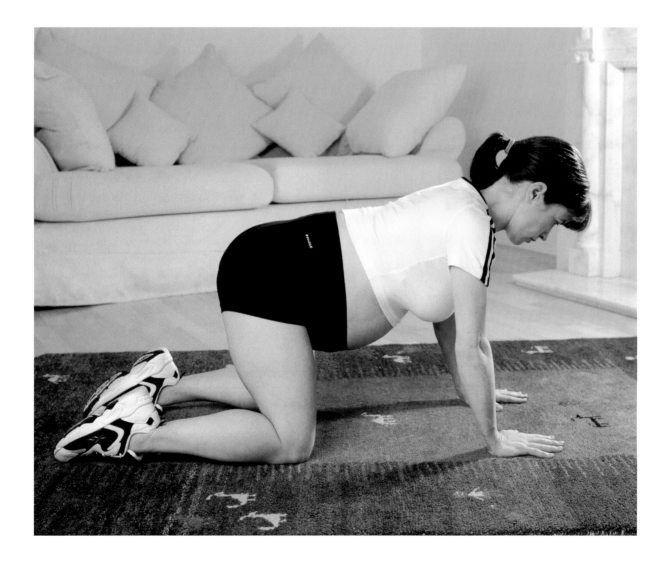

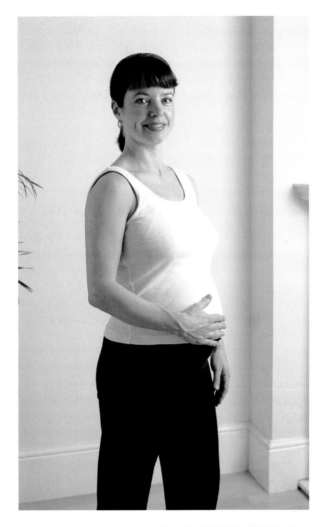

Posture

Maintaining correct posture throughout your pregnancy can help to get your tummy flat again after childbirth. As your baby grows, you will need to adjust your posture to take account of your growing baby, it's effect on the abdominal corset, and your changing centre of gravity. Correct posture shifts your weight so that it is evenly supported by your skeleton, rather than putting undue strain on any one part. This relieves the strain of the excess load off your tummy and back.

Good posture in pregnancy
- Stand tall with shoulders relaxed
- Keep your lower back in a neutral position (not arched)
- Keep your pelvis tucked in
- Hold your tummy tight so that your ribs are a little in front of and lifted up from your baby.

Look at yourself in a mirror in profile every month of your pregnancy to check that you are maintaining correct posture If you're not sure, ask a qualified exercise instructor.

What is a diastasis?

A diastasis occurs when the separation of the two halves of the rectus abdominus muscle that occurs during pregnancy do not go back after pregnancy. You can check for it by lying on your back with your knees bent. (If you start to feel faint on your back, roll to your left side, and use pillows under your shoulders to prop yourself up.) Place your fingertips one to two inches below your belly button, fingers pointing toward your feet. Lift your head up and forward, eyes looking in front of you. Can you feel a ridge protruding from the midline of your abdomen? That's a diastasis. If you have it, take care not to make the separation worse by doing abdominal exercises on your back.

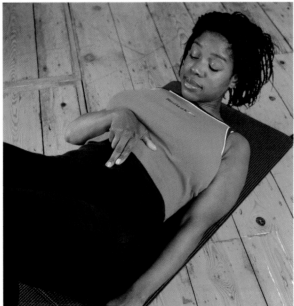

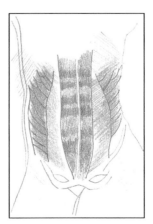

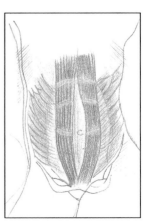

figure 4. Normal muscles. *figure 5. A diastasis.*

Your skin

During pregnancy, your uterus expands above your navel and your abdomen stretches to accommodate it. On average, a pregnant woman's skin stretches from 17 to 18.5 square feet by the time she's ready to deliver, and most of this expansion is on her tummy. To ensure that the skin on your tummy regains it's tone, you need to treat it.

Our skin is our waterproof covering, we do not absorb bath water or thick mineral oils like petroleum jelly, which leaves a thick greasy layer on the skin. But it is possible for the skin to allow through certain substances if their molecular structure is small enough.

The skin is one of the body's organs of elimination. We lose sweat and other soluble wastes through our skin and so in the same way it lets things out, we can let things in. Doctors are now increasingly administering medications, such as anti-angina and HRT by applying them to the skin, which means they bypass the digestive system and, in turn, are kinder to the body's internal organs.

When applied to the skin, a hydrating oil such as jojoba or wheatgerm and aromatherapy oils have tiny molecular structures that enable them to pass through the skin. They travel via the hair follicles, diffusing into the bloodstream, or as lymphatic and extra-cellular fluids. It is here at cellular level that the oils and essential oils are broken down and used to hydrate the skin.

Jojoba oil
Jojoba oil is probably the most important skin care item to keep the skin on your tummy, and anywhere else, supple and elastic. It can help prevent stretch marks, and help the skin to spring back after childbirth.

The oil from jojoba seeds is very similar in nature and acid balance (pH) to sebum, the oil naturally secreted by human sebaceous glands. Sebum protects and moisturises the skin and hair, but it is stripped away by chemicals, pollutants, the sun and age, resulting in dry skin and hair. Pure jojoba oil replenishes what our skin and hair loses, and restores their natural balance.

Starting from our early 20s (even younger if we spend a lot of time in the sun), our skin starts to lose its elasticity. It cracks with the progressive loss of elastin, the protein that keeps skin flexible and moist. Oils contain insaponifiables, and these substances, when applied to the skin maintain the condition of elastin. Most vegetable oils about 2-3% insaponifiables – Jojoba has 50%.

Essential oils
Massaging skin with essential oils can restore suppleness. These essential oils need to be mixed with a base oil such as jojoba or wheatgerm oil, and massaged into the skin.

- Fennel oil contains phytomones which can firm skin and stimulate cell metabolism.
- Lavender can help fade stretch marks.
- Neroli can speed up cell replacement
- Patchouli can help cell renewal
- Echinacea does not come in an essential oil form, but is thought to stimulate collagen and elastin. The tincture would need to be added to a base cream.

Retinol
Retinol is plain old Vitamin A. The benefits of retinol in skincare were discovered when acne patients were treated with retinoic acid, a caustic derivative of vitamin A, and lost not only their spots, but also their wrinkles.

Researchers observed that retinol cream repaired damaged skin tissue, promoted the growth of healthy new collagen, smoothed out roughness, and reduced the appearance of sun-induced blemishes such as age spots. In other words, retinol improved the skin in all the areas that differentiates old from young skin.

A retinol based cream used on the tummy may help to smooth out surplus wrinkly skin, but it is doubtful that it can restore very stretched skin to it's original taut state. Retinol based products are not recommended for Black, Asian or Olive skins.

Vitamin C
Vitamin C plays an essential role in every aspect of the skin's functioning including growth, repair of connective tissue, protection from free radical oxidation damage, wound healing, collagen synthesis, and prevention of premature ageing.

Collagen constitutes 80% of the dermis (outer layer of the skin), and the collagen structures that support the skin maintain a firm foundation that retains tautness.

Under clinical laboratory conditions, scientists were able to cause collagen synthesis as well as stimulate cell rejuvenation by transporting Vitamin C into cells.

The Waist

7

(Your Skin continued.)

MSM

MSM stands for Methyl Sulphonyl Methane. It is a naturally occurring nutrient, and organic sulphur compound that is found in the normal human diet. Sulphur is present in all living organisms, and helps to maintain the structure of the body's proteins.

There has been anecdotal evidence that MSM may reduce the extent of cross-linking in the collagen and elastin fibres of the skin. Since cross-linking causes wrinkle formation, MSM may help to delay or reduce wrinkle formation.

Salon treatments

The claim for many salon treatments is that they can firm skin and fade stretch marks whilst you lose subcutaneous fat and tone muscles.

Treatments such as CACI, Ionithermie, and Gatineau use a combination of massage, electrical stimuli, ultrasound, thermal clay and algae treatments. Of all the salon treatments we tested, Arasys got the best results (for more details see page 91).

It is important to ask to see your beautician's qualifications, check that the salon is adequately insured, and make sure that there is a high standard of hygiene before undergoing your treatment

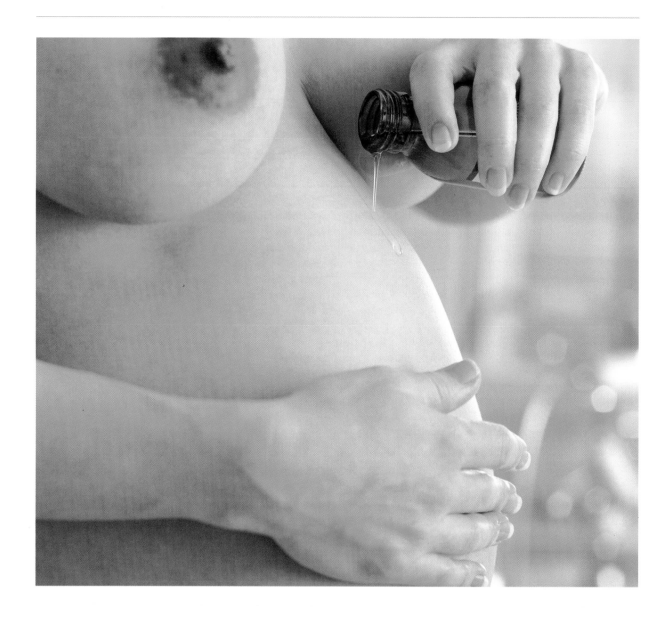

How do you turn a 'baby belly' into a flat stomach?

Watching daytime television one morning, I listened to a phone-in where women discussed the parts of their bodies they were least happy with. Someone phoned in saying that she hated her tummy, which was flabby with loose skin after having had two children. She was advised by one of the 'experts' on the panel that this protruding stomach after childbirth was 'stubborn fat', almost impossible to get rid of, and that the most effective and quickest way to get rid of it was an abdominoplasty, or 'tummy tuck.'

To say that I was shocked to hear such advice was an understatement. A tummy tuck is a major surgical procedure that produces a permanent scar that can extend from hip to hip.

Fat will go off the body with a combination of good nutrition and the right sort of fat burning exercises. You cannot pick the spot that you want to reduce. Ignore diets that claim that you can reduce fat specifically from your hips and thighs or anywhere else. Fat goes off the body in the same sequence no matter what plan you use.

The good news is that the tummy is one of the first places that it will go from. Fat goes first from the abdominal cavity, then from the face, then from between the shoulder blades, and then from the hips and thighs.

So how do you get a flat stomach? Sit-ups, sit-ups, and more sit-ups? No! Not in our programme. We all have flat stomachs most of us have 'six packs'. The problem is that they are hidden beneath a layer of fat. Doing sit-ups and crunches may strengthen your abdominals, but unless you get rid of that layer of fat, your flat stomach will not show. If I had been on that expert panel, Here's what I would have told the lady who was advised to have a tummy tuck.

Five steps to a tight tummy
1. Cut all saturated fats out of your diet. That's not all fats, just saturated fats that are found in butter, cheese, egg yolks, chicken, beef, lamb and pork chops, biscuits and cakes. This still leaves plenty of choice. You just need to be careful to cut the fat off all the meat you eat, and take the skin off chicken. You can have stir fries with olive oil and lots of vegetables, and can eat fish such as salmon and tuna, where you will get a good supply of healthy fish oils. Also get a daily serving of flax seed oil as you need fat to burn fat (see Chapter 6).

2. Eat low fat proteins such as skinless chicken breast, egg white omelettes, tofu, and skimmed milk (see Chapter 6).

3. Eat lots of slow burning carbohydrates and cut down on the fast burners. Have porridge oats instead of cornflakes, wholemeal pitta bread instead of sliced white bread, basmati rice, wholewheat pasta, and lots of vegetables. Have these complex carbohydrate meals earlier in the day rather than later as they help sustain energy levels, and have your dinner before seven. Try to eat some protein with every meal, even if it's some tofu mixed in with your pasta (see Chapter 6).

4. Do some kind of aerobic exercise, preferably walking, as it is low impact, and will use fat as an energy source (see Chapter 3).

5. Adopt a strength training programme (see Chapter 2), and include the abdominal exercises described later in the chapter. Strength training has a dramatic effect on the fat on your tummy. This is thought to be because fat cells in the abdominal area release their contents for energy utilisation far more readily than fat cells in the thighs and buttocks which are used for long-term energy storage. Also, whereas aerobic exercise reduces subcutaneous fat (fat under the skin), strength training reduces the excess fat around internal organs which adds to belly fat.

If you follow these steps, you will quickly notice results. As your abdominals become tightened, the loose skin in the area may also tighten up as well, though it needs to be nourished to help it regain elasticity. There may be some stretch marks left, but with time these may fade.

7

The Exercises
During Pregnancy

1. Pelvic floor muscles

In pregnancy, the pelvic floor is usually able to stretch more in preparation for delivery which with the weight of the baby, may weaken the muscles. This can cause stress incontinence, you can wet yourself if you cough, sneeze or move quickly. Do these pelvic floor exercises (called Kegel exercises after the doctor who developed them) as often as you can, even if you are not pregnant yet. You can be in any position sitting, standing or lying. Think about trying to draw up and close your back passage (anus) as if to stop yourself from passing wind. Draw up and close your front passage as if to stop the flow of urine. Squeeze and lift up inside the vagina. Hold the squeeze for a few seconds then let go slowly. Don't hold your breath when you are squeezing. Try to increase the length of the squeeze up to 10 seconds. Repeat up to 10 times an hour. Once you are comfortable with this technique, try doing some quick one-second contractions as well as the long hold ones.

2. Tummy contractions

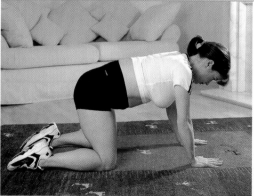

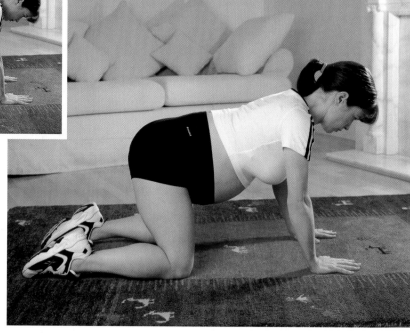

Kneel on all fours, keeping your hands in line with your shoulders. Contract your abs so that your spine is in a flat (not arched) position (see picture right). Keeping your back straight and flat, contract your stomach muscles and lift your baby up and in towards your spine (see above). Hold for a count of five, counting out loud to ensure that you are not holding your breath. Slowly release, taking care not to allow your back to sag. The weight of the baby gives your muscles an excellent workout.

3. Cat stretch

In the same position as for the tummy contraction, contract your abs so that your spine is in a flat position. Stretch your shoulders. Squeeze your buttocks and bring your pelvis under you. Curl your head forward and down for a count of eight. Release gently, taking care not to allow your back to sag. Repeat for two sets of six to eight repetions. (If your wrists are sore, rest on your arms forward on the seat of a sturdy chair.)

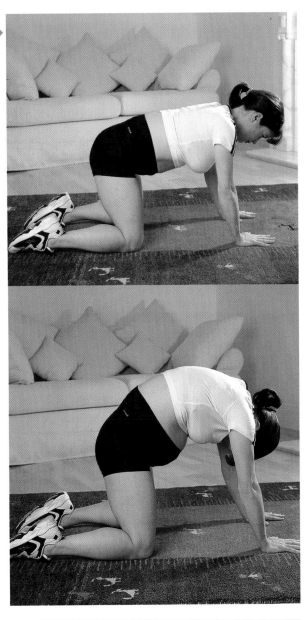

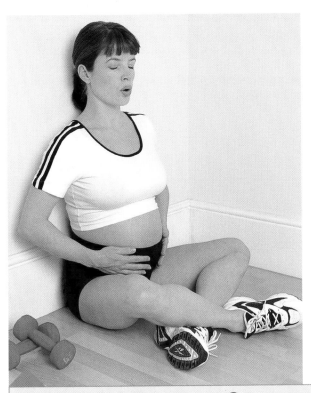

4. Seated Tummy Contractions

Sit cross-legged against a support that makes contact with your entire back. Put your hands on your belly to feel the abdominal contractions. Breathe in and expand your belly. As you breathe out slowly, concentrate on contracting your abs inwards. Hold for a count of five, and release. Repeat six to eight times.

5. Holding your tummy in

The most important abdominal exercise, which can be done at any time and should be done at all times. It is simply holding your tummy in. Do a posture check, tuck your pelvis under, and contract your stomach muscles. Again think of it as pulling your baby towards you.

7

First six weeks after childbirth

You can start within hours of delivery with simply pulling in your abdominal muscles imagine that you are trying to get into a really tight pair of jeans.

If you have had a caesarean section, before you get out of bed, try to wiggle your toes, flex your calves, bend your feet up at the ankles, push against the end of the bed with your feet, and turn your body from side to side. These exercises are intended to improve circulation, especially in your legs to prevent blood clots. (Be prepared to feel some pain or feel sore for the first three to four days.) When you feel ready you can also start the following exercises.

1. Belly breathing

Lie on your back in bed or on the floor. Bend your knees and keep your feet flat. Breathe in and expand your abdomen. Contract your muscles as tightly as you can, pulling your navel towards your spine. At the same time, tilt your pelvis back, bringing your hips towards your lower ribs. Begin with as many as you can do, building up to 15 a day. When you can do 15 repetitions, begin to lift your head, neck and shoulders up with each contraction.

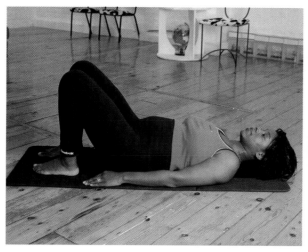 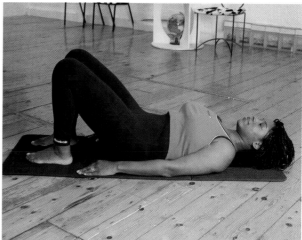

2. Standing stomach vacuum

This is the same exercise as above except from the standing position. It is best done first thing in the morning, before breakfast. Slightly bend your knees and place a hand on each knee. Breathe out and vacuum in your stomach, then release. Try to hold for the count of 8. Work yourself up to 8-10 repetitions.

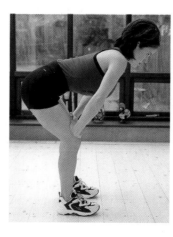 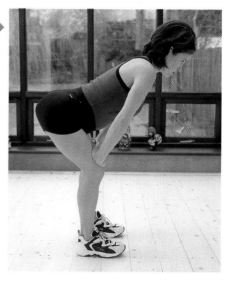

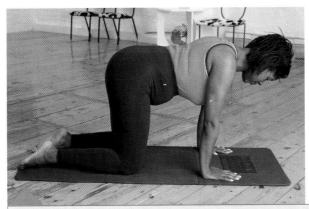 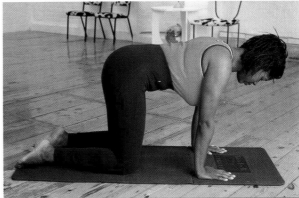

3. Tummy contractions

Kneel on all fours, keep your hands in line with your shoulders. Contract your abdominals so that your spine is in a flat position. Keeping your back straight and flat, contract your tummy muscles and pull in towards your spine. Hold for the count of five, count out loud to ensure you are not holding your breath and slowly release, taking care not to let your back sag.

4. Cat stretch

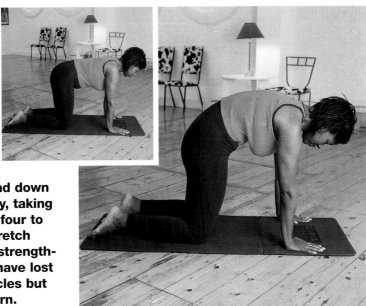

Cat stretches are perhaps the most important of the realignment exercises. Kneel on all fours, keep your hands in line with your shoulders. Contract your abdominals so that your spine is in a flat position (not arched). Stretch your shoulders. Squeeze your buttocks and pelvic tilt. Curl your head forward and down for the count of eight. Release gently, taking care not to arch the back. Do about four to six of each type. These exercises stretch your back muscles, and also gently strengthen your abs. You may feel as if you have lost all feeling with your abdominal muscles but stick with it and the feeling will return.

5. Holding your tummy in

Equally important, this is the most straightforward exercise, but also the hardest to remember. Dancers and ballerinas do it all the time, that is why they have such good posture. Holding your stomach in re-establishes your abdominal posture, also it reminds you to keep good posture in your back as well. Stand tall, lifting yourself from the waist, elongating your spine, tuck your pelvis under and breath in your tummy, hold the muscles tight and release. Try to do this as often as possible eventually you will constantly hold your tummy tight without even realising it.

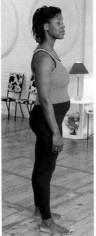 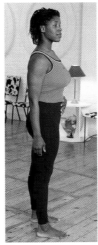

| Bad posture with tummy out | Good posture with tummy out | Good posture with tummy in |

7

After the six week check

(and only if less than a two finger width gap between
the rectus abdominus when checking for separation)

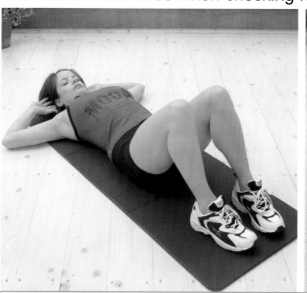 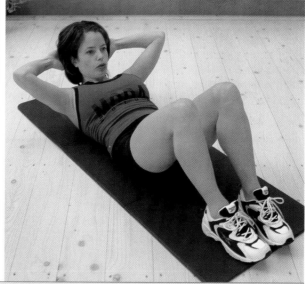

1. Basic crunch see below

Lie on your back, with your knees bent and shoulder width apart. Place your hands on the
tops of your thighs, arms fully extended. Your chin should be about a fist's distance from
your chest. As you curl upwards,
imagine curling one vertebra off the
floor at a time. Keep your head,
neck, and arms frozen in position.
They play no role in the exercise
your abs should do the work. As you
curl, tighten your abs and then
breathe out forcefully though your
mouth. As you lower your torso,
keep your abs tight and breathe in
deeply through your nose. Try to do
two sets of 12 repetitions.

2. Extended crunch
see above

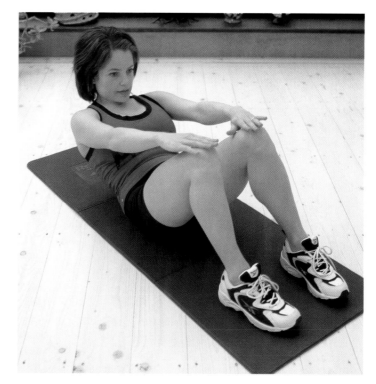

Start as for the basic crunch.
This time place your hands behind
your head but do not lace your fingers. Breathing out, slowly curl
yourself up. Hold for a count of five
at the peak of the movement then
slowly uncurl. Try to work yourself
up to two sets of 12 repetitions.

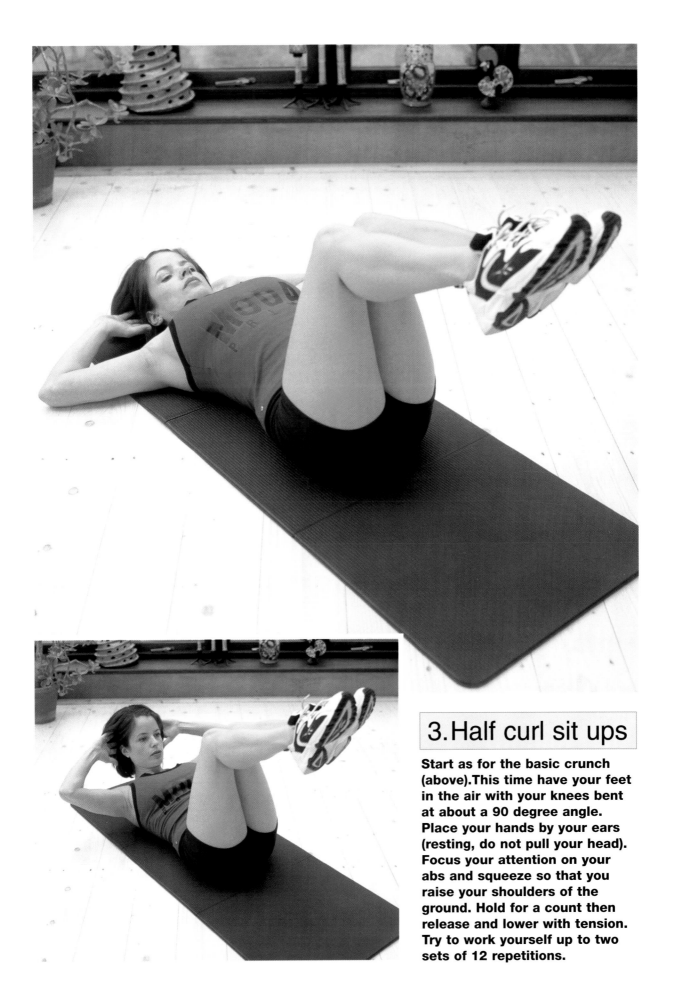

3. Half curl sit ups

Start as for the basic crunch
(above).This time have your feet
in the air with your knees bent
at about a 90 degree angle.
Place your hands by your ears
(resting, do not pull your head).
Focus your attention on your
abs and squeeze so that you
raise your shoulders of the
ground. Hold for a count then
release and lower with tension.
Try to work yourself up to two
sets of 12 repetitions.

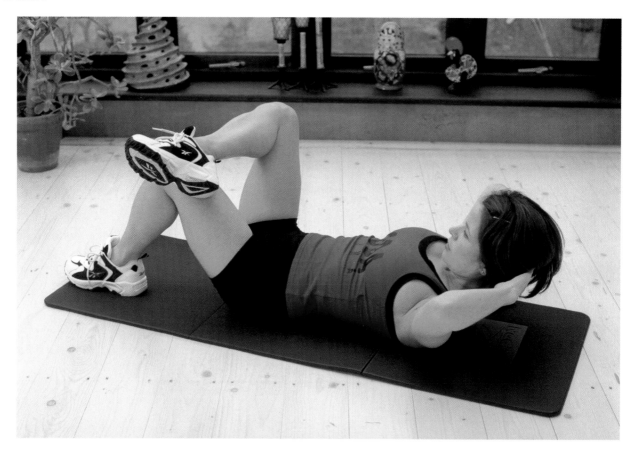

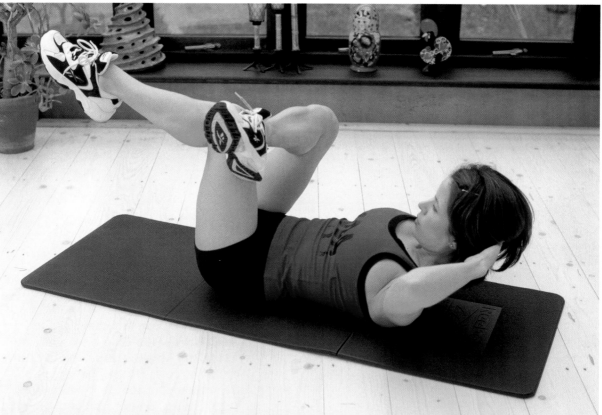

4. Single leg half raises

Lie on your back as in basic crunch, with knees bent and shoulder width apart. Bend your right knee and place your left foot on your right knee. Place your hands on either side of your head and lift your head and shoulders off the ground. This is your starting position. Lift your right foot off the ground about 30cm and return. Repeat 10 times then change legs.

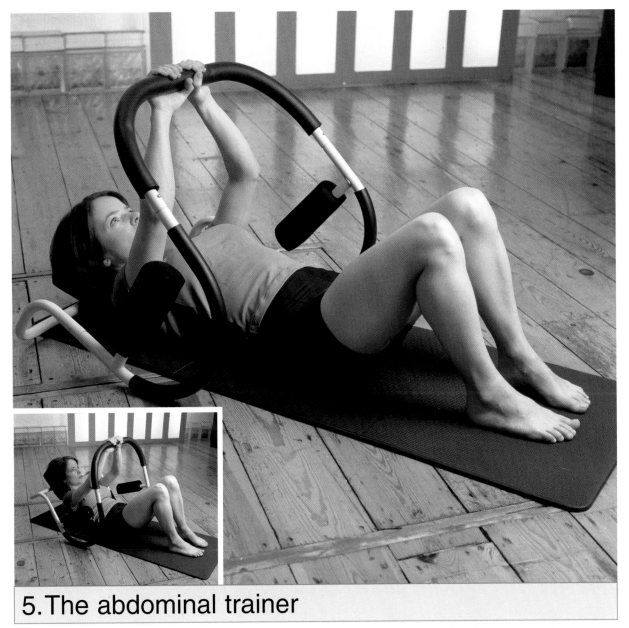

5. The abdominal trainer

The abdominal trainer helps to concentrate the workout to the abdominal area to improve the waistline and strengthen the tummy muscles. It prevents you placing any strain on the back, neck, and head. To work the abdominal area efficiently, it is best to keep your head and neck locked in position – the padded cushion on the cage helps you achieve this.

Electrical stimulation

If you find abdominal exercises tedious (I know that many do), you could try following the five steps and use electrical stimulation on the abdominal area.

Electrical stimulation enables you to work a particular muscle many more times than you would otherwise. Unlike other muscle groups which you need to rest, you can work the abdominals every day.

I tried electrical stimulation in an attempt to get rid of my baby belly, and it did help. Because I had a wide diastasis on my abdominal muscles, a lot of abdominal exercises would have made it worse.

The Arasys system was designed by scientists at the South Bank University in London. Each 17 minute session can do the equivalent of 300 crunches. Arasys made a difference from the second session and I certainly believe it is effective toning.

Home systems such as Ultratone work along the same principles but beware of cheaper versions which generate sudden, jerky muscle movements..

Electrical stimulation helps to tone the muscles, but it is important that you complement it with lots of walking and some strength training to help rid the fat from the tummy.

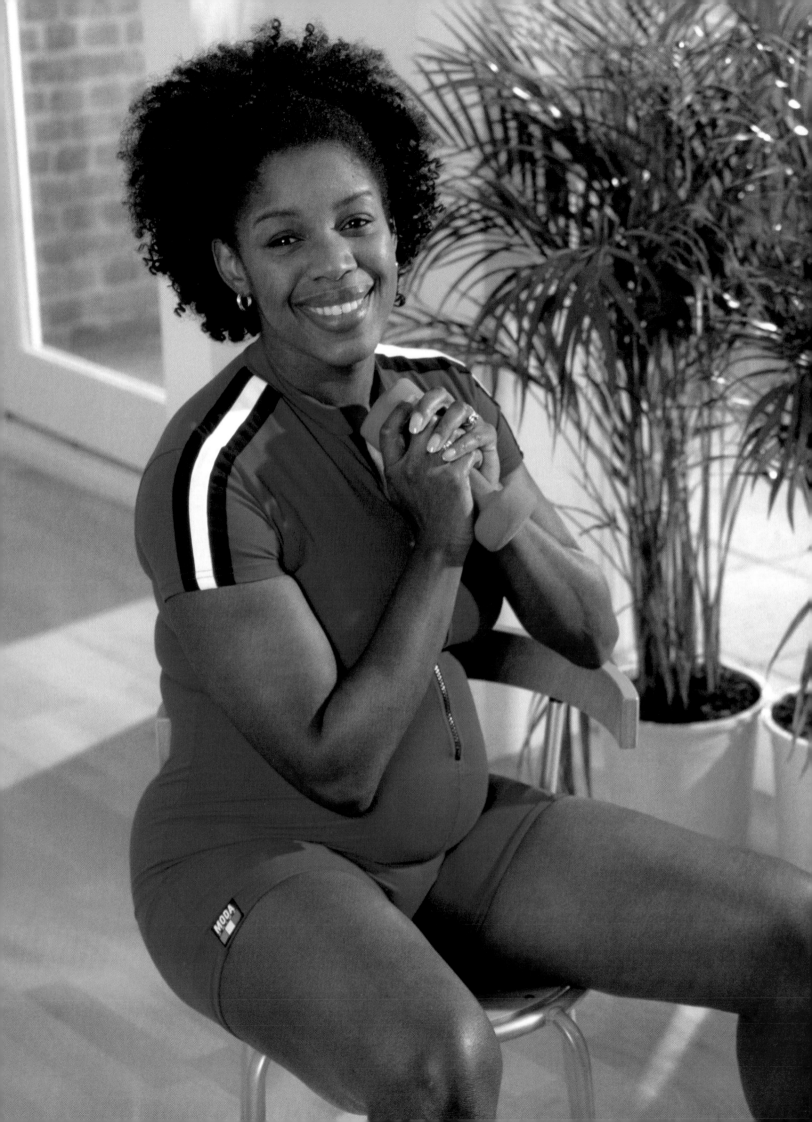

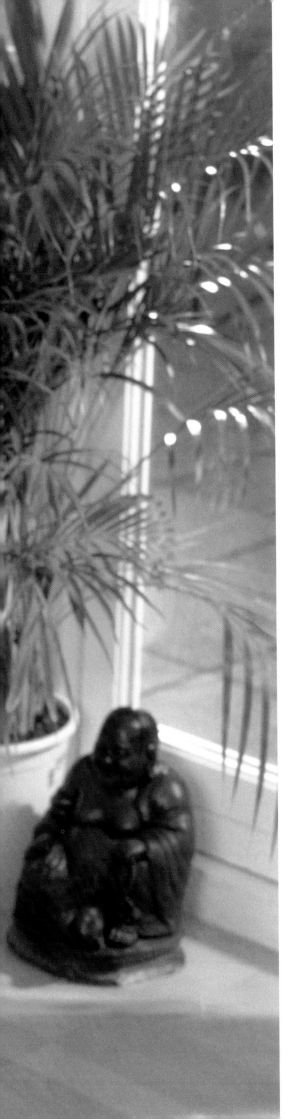

Exercises During Pregnancy

When a woman gives birth, she must summon the strength and stamina of an elite athlete. With the muscle activity of the uterus, childbirth is chiefly a muscular action, so it makes sense to train for the event.

This programme combines two types of exercise for maximum benefits:
Strength training will help you meet the huge physical demands of pregnancy.
Aerobic conditioning will give you the stamina for pregnancy, labour and birth.

The programme has three levels of fitness.
Choose Level One:
if you're a beginner and are just starting to exercise
Choose Level Two:
if you have regularly exercised once or twice a week; or
if you have been at Level One for about a month
Choose Level Three:
if you have exercised regularly three times per week;
or if you have been at Level Two for about a month

Each strength training workout takes about 15-20 minutes. You should do one aerobic conditioning workout for every strength training workout. Aim for three sessions of each per week in the first trimester, and two or three sessions of each in the second and third trimester. The strength training workout incorporates just the very basic exercises, but it covers all the main muscle groups, and will make you stronger.

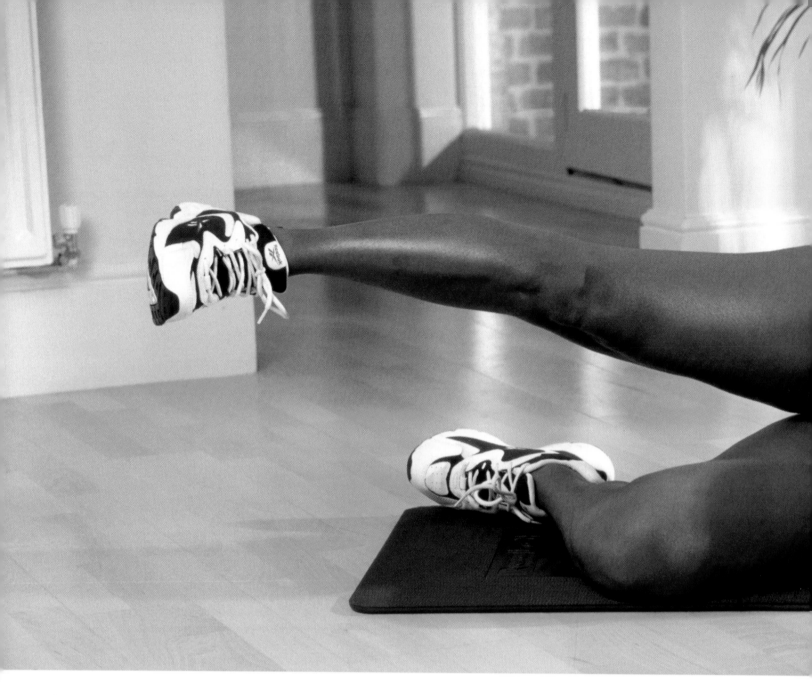

Starting off

Remember to listen to your body. If your body says 'no' to exercise, don't force it. Start off with gentle walking and then try to add more exercises. Begin each routine at a gentle pace, gradually building up to what feels right for you. Concentrate on getting the full benefits from each exercise by going through each exercise slowly and deliberately. If you simply swing the dumbbells, you will not gain any benefits and you may injure yourself. Quality of movement is all important. Strength training works because you are isolating each particular muscle with control.

Breathing

Getting your breathing right is vital to strength training. It may help to take some deep breaths after warming up and before you start each exercise. Exhale on the lift part of the move that requires the effort. Inhale as you go back to the starting position. Never hold your breath while doing any exercise.

The wrists

Oedema associated with pregnancy can cause swelling in the wrists (carpel tunnel syndrome, see page 98), so we have avoided exercises that flex the wrists.

When to stop

If you experience any of the following, stop exercising immediately:

● **Pain of any kind (seek medical advice)**
● **Faintness or dizziness**
● **Fatigue – do not exercise to exhaustion**
● **Braxton Hicks contractions**
● **Cramping (gently stretch out the affected part)**
● **Shortness of breath (take slow deep breaths)**

When you resume, do so at a slower pace and lifting gentler weights.

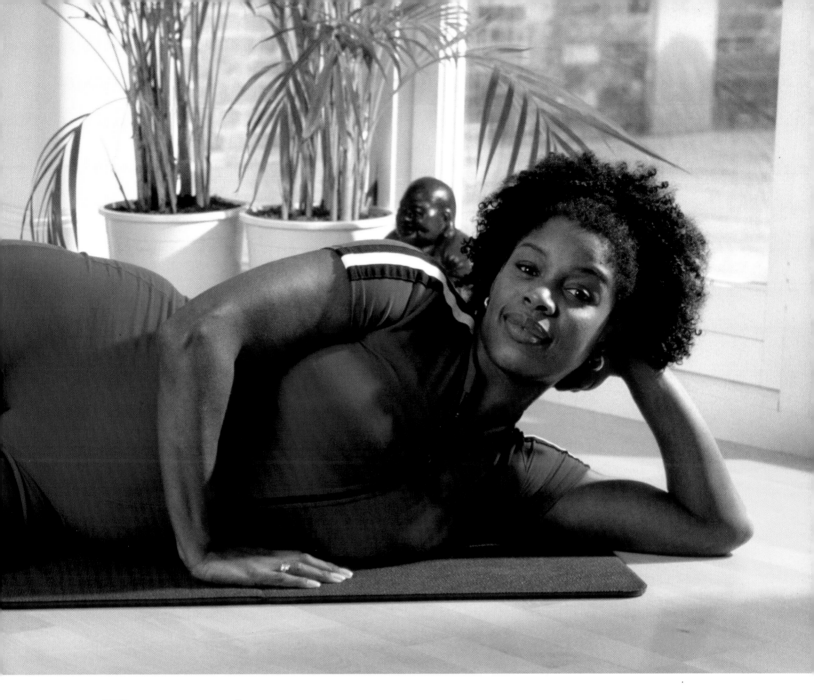

The muscle groups

We have devised the programme to exercise the muscle groups that need to be strong during pregnancy. They are:

● Pectoral (chest) muscles
● Abdominal (tummy) muscles
● Leg muscles
● Shoulder and arm muscles
● Back muscles

Pectorals

The extra weight of larger breasts during pregnancy can pull the shoulders forward, shortening the pectoral muscles in the chest on which the breasts sit. This can stress the rhomboid and trapezius muscles in the upper back. Strengthening the pecs will tighten the tissue supporting the breasts and help you to maintain your shape.

Abdominals

If your abdominal muscles are weak, the added weight of your baby will pull your posture forward and curve your back causing lower back pain. Strong abdominal muscles will support your pregnant tummy, improve your posture, and strengthen your back. They will also help you to get your waist back after you have had your baby (see Chapter 7).

Legs

Strong legs enable you to carry your extra weight comfortably and confidently. You may also suffer fewer leg cramps and swelling.

Shoulders and arms

Carrying a baby around takes more strength and endurance than you think. Strong shoulders and arms will prevent some of the aches and pains of motherhood. Strong shoulders also help posture.

Back

A strong back can help prevent the back pains associated with pregnancy. It also completes the strong girdle of muscles supporting your baby.

What you will need

For the strength training exercises you will need just a set of dumbbells. It may be a good idea to buy dumbbells with varying weights. You could also use tins of beans or soup. Walking shoes are also necessary for this exercise pro-gramme.

What weights to use (weights are in kilograms)

	1st trimester	2nd trimester	3rd trimester
Level 1	2	2	1
Level 2	up to 5	3	2
Level 3	5 or above	up to 5	3 or less

The important thing is to lift the weight that you are comfort-able with. Even if you are very fit and strong, do not use too heavy a weight because of the risk of spraining due to the effect of relaxin on the joints. It is better to increase repeti-tions rather than weight.

Be sure to store your dumbbells in a safe place when you're not using them.

Aerobic exercises

Walking is one of the best ways to exercise your heart and lungs in pregnancy.

Walking

● is low impact and does not stress the joints or the fetus
● is fat burning
● works the large muscles in your legs and buttocks.

Walking is the most straightforward exercise. It costs noth-ing, you get plenty of fresh air, and a good pair of walking shoes or trainers is all the equipment you need.

The real beauty of it is that when you're ready to ease back into exercise after the baby, you can just put your new arrival in a push-chair, or strap her to your chest, and off you go.

To improve cardiovascular fitness during pregnancy, it is better to increase the duration of your walk while maintain-ing or reducing your intensity (speed and incline). A long gentle stroll is better than a short power walk, especially in the third trimester.

No matter how fit you were pre-pregnancy, you must expect to do less as pregnancy progresses. The third trimester especially is not a time to do anything that you are not used to.

Some tips on walking during pregnancy

● **Listen to your body. Focus on how you feel. You may have more energy one day and can try walking a little more. On other days you may be feeling tired so slow down and take a break. When your body says stop, STOP.**

● **Find a walking partner this makes walking a lot more fun.**

● **Use the talk test. If you can't carry on a conversation while you're walking, you are walking too fast. Slow down. You should feel slightly short of breath but able to talk.**

● **Walk tall with your chest and shoulders lifted, hold your tummy in. This will lessen the arch in your back from the extra weight in front.**

● **Tilt your pelvis – this will keep your spine correctly aligned and prevent you from sticking your bottom out (which compounds backache).**

● **Imagine that you're trying to spread your ribs. This will make more room in the diaphragm and make breathing easier.**

● **Take small steps – as your belly grows, a shorter stride will help you keep your centre of gravity squarely beneath you and you won't lose your balance.**

● **Land heel first, and let your foot roll naturally through to push off with the ball of your foot.**

● **Swing your arms, though not wildly. This will give you a better aerobic workout. Hold your hands in loose fists.**

● **Dress in layers, and be careful not to overheat, especially in the first trimester.**

● **Do not wear a tight bra: this will restrict the diaphragm, restrict your breathing, and you may feel faint.**

● **Drink plenty of water before, during and after your workout.**

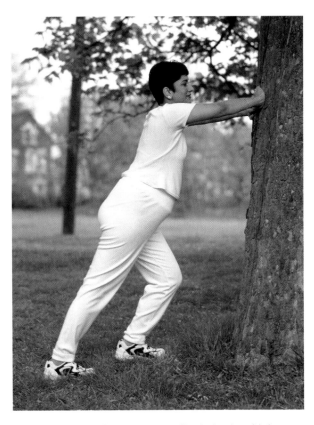

Warm up

Before each walk, be sure to warm up. Begin each walk at an easy pace for five minutes, then stop to stretch your calves.

Cool down

When you're coming to the end of your walk, slow down to warm up pace for at least five minutes. Then stretch your calves and while holding a support, stretch your hip flexors by holding one foot at a time behind your back. Hold each stretch for 30 to 40 seconds without bouncing (leave this out if you find it difficult).

We don't want to set a walking programme, because all throughout this book we are saying to listen to your body, and respond to the messages it sends you.

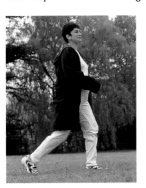

What we will say is follow the tips on walking during pregnancy, and walk for as long as you are comfortable. I was quite fit before my pregnancy, but by the third trimester I could not walk for longer than 15 minutes. Tonia however, was not very fit before her first pregnancy but was still going for hour long walks during her third trimester.

This illustrates how subjective each pregnancy is. If you can only manage five minutes, that's okay. Never push yourself. Your body knows best, listen to it. If you are walking on a treadmill, do not use an inclined treadmill as this puts too much pressure on the back.

Other aerobic exercises for pregnancy

Swimming

Swimming and water exercises are good while pregnant because the water takes your weight, while offering good resistance so that your muscles get a good workout. Also swimming is a good relaxation exercise. Go to the pool at a quiet time and just float, or try your local pool for antenatal classes.

Stationary cycling

A recumbent cycling machine is the best stationary cycling to use when pregnant because it allows for the easier accommodation of an expanding girth.

Aerobic Exercises that require more care (see Chapter 7 – The Waist for explanations):

● Step and bench aerobics
● Jogging
● High Impact aerobics

Maximum heart rate

We have not given maximum heart rate recommendations as the use of heart rate to assess exercise intensity is inaccurate during pregnancy. It tends to give higher training values.

See Chapter 9 for heart rate guidelines after childbirth.

Strength exercises
Precautions for exercise during pregnancy

Carpal tunnel syndrome

This mainly occurs during the third trimester, it is a numbing of the thumb, index, middle and half of the ring fingers. The carpal tunnel is in the wrist and the nerve for these fingers runs through it. During pregnancy it can become swollen, (as do many other tissues in the body) but the resultant pressure causes numbness, tingling or pain. Because of this we have mainly avoided exercises where too much weight is put on the hands. If numbness does occur, try taking hands up to shoulder height and rotating the wrists.

Symphysis pubis (part of the pubic bone)

The symphysis pubis has a pad of cartilage between the two joint surfaces of the pubic bones and plays an important role in the stability of the pelvis. It is also dependent on ligaments which are affected by relaxin during pregnancy. This can cause it to become a source of discomfort, therefore avoid any exercises that need wide leg separation if you have any kind of discomfort

Supine hypotensive syndrome

Reduced venous return is most pronounced when lying flat on the back where the pregnant uterus presses on the inferior vena cava, the great vein which takes all the blood from the abdomen and legs back to the heart. This can cause a reduction in cardiac output and lead to dizziness or even a loss of consciousness. It may even interfere with blood flow to the fetus. It can be relieved by lying slightly on one side, especially the right side.

Postural hypotensive syndrome

Progesterone causes reduced vascular resistance and vein wall tone. This reduces venous return from your legs. You should avoid standing still for too long as this allows blood to pool in your legs and can cause faintness. Movement promotes venous return as the calf muscles squeeze the blood through the veins and back to your heart.

Stretches

Stretching during pregnancy is very important, but because of the effects of relaxin in your system you must be careful not to over-extend your stretch, as this may cause joint instability. Stretching helps prevent stiffness, keeps your body supple and lessens the risk of muscle injury and cramp.

1. Side stretch

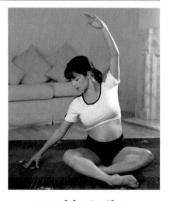

Sit comfortably on the floor. Lean to the side with your right hand on the floor for support. Straighten your left arm overhead and bend over your right. Keep the top arm slightly forward and bottom firmly on the floor, and shoulders square. Turn your chin to the right and glance down. You should feel a continuous stretch down your left side. Tighten your tummy muscles and lift through the back. Hold a comfortable stretch for 10-20 seconds, return to centre. Change legs and repeat on other side.

2. Head and neck roll

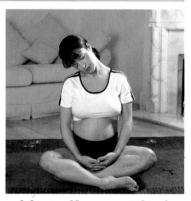

Sit tall on the edge of a sturdy chair, knees bent and feet flat on the floor about hip width apart. Or sit cross-legged. Let your head hang forward relaxing the nape of the neck, shoulders and face. Keep your back straight. Focus your attention on your breathing. Slowly turn your head from side to side, while breathing deeply.

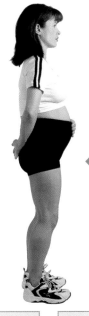

The warm-up

This is a good time to look at your posture. This is very important both during and after pregnancy. Poor posture pulls the body out of alignment and leads to additional strain on the back and supporting muscles. During pregnancy the baby's weight pulls you forward, which results in a tendency to lean back to compensate, thus causing backache.

1. Posture check

Relax your shoulders and gently press them down. Lift your chest and ribs. Tighten your tummy and tilt your pelvis gently under. Keep your back straight and relax your knees. This is known as holding your spine in a neutral position.

2. Squat spring

Stand firmly with feet facing forward and shoulder width apart. Gently bend knees into a quarter squat, swinging arms forward and up, lowering down to sides as the legs straighten. Keeping tummy tight and pelvis tilted under. Repeat 8-10 times or until you begin to feel warm.

3. Ceiling stretch

Stand with feet slightly wider than shoulders, place one hand on hip. Check your pelvis is straight and tilted, tummy tight. Reach one arm up to the ceiling, lengthening and extending the spine. Hold, then slowly come down and repeat with the other arm. Keep the arm slightly forward to prevent the back arching.

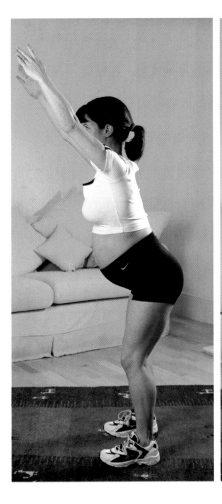
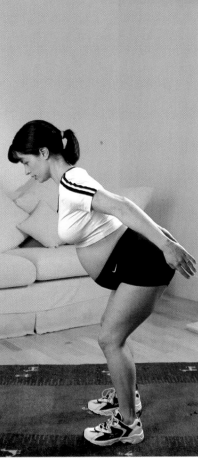
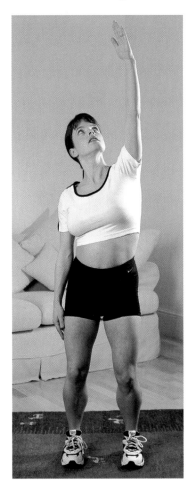

8

Abdomen and back
Abdominals (Refer to Chapter 7)

1. Tummy contraction

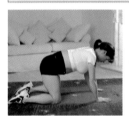

Kneel on all fours, keep your hands in line with your shoulders. Contract abdominals so that your spine is in neutral position (not arched). Keeping back straight and flat, contract your stomach muscles and lift your baby up and in towards your spine. Hold for a count of five; count out loud to ensure you are not holding your breath and slowly release, taking care not to allow the back to arch. Repeat for two sets of six to eight repetitions. The weight of the baby gives your muscles an excellent workout.

2. Cat stretch

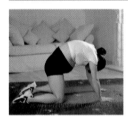

In the same position, contract abdominals so that your spine is in neutral position; relax your shoulders. Squeeze your buttocks and bring your pelvis under you. Curl your head forward and down for a count of eight. Release gently, taking care not to allow the back to arch. Repeat for two sets of six to eight repetitions. (If wrists are sore, rest on your arms forward on the seat of a sturdy chair.)

3. Seated tummy contraction

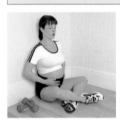

Sit against a support that makes contact with your entire back. It is good to put your hands on your belly to feel the abdominal contractions. Inhale and expand your belly, slowly exhale, concentrate on contracting your abdominals inwards. Hold for a count of 5 and slowly release. Repeat for two sets of eight repetitions.

4. Holding your tummy in

The most important abdominal exercise, which can be done anytime and should be done at all times. It is simply holding your tummy in. Check your posture, tuck your pelvis under, and contract your stomach muscles, again think of it as pulling your baby towards you.

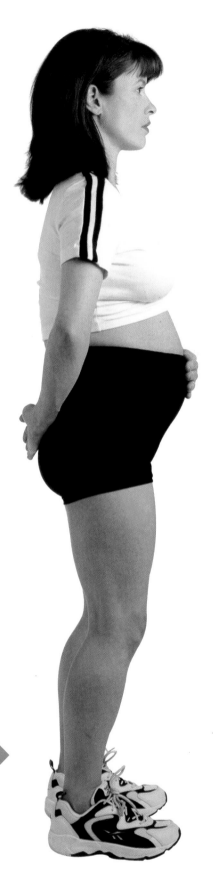

Back

1.Upper back stretch

Sit cross-legged or sit tall on the edge of a sturdy chair, knees bent and feet flat on the floor about hip width apart. Raise your arm up and across your chest. Support your arm just above the elbow with your other hand and gently ease it towards your body. Keeping shoulders relaxed, and the back lifted, hold for 10 to 20 seconds. Repeat with other arm.

2.Single arms rows

Stand with one foot in front of the other with a wide base, and support yourself with one hand on the back of a high chair. Posture check. Hold a dumbbell in one hand and in bent over position, fully extend the arm forward and down, but do not allow the elbow to lock. Keep the arm facing forward, and the wrist in line with the forearm, bring the elbow back. Repeat 12 times on each side.

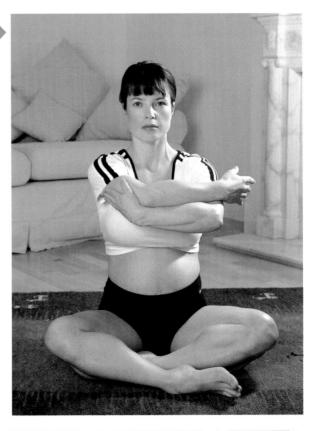

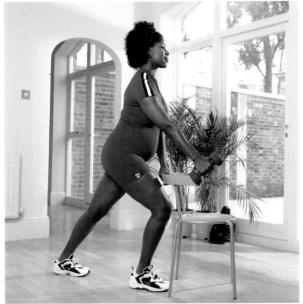

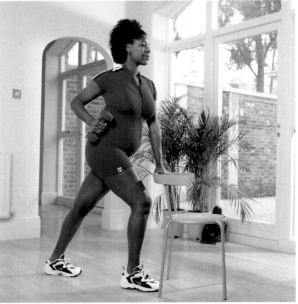

3.Repeat upper back stretch

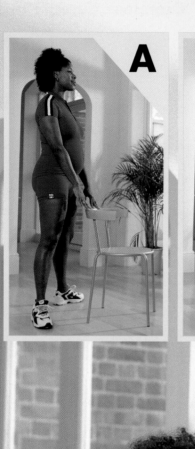

A

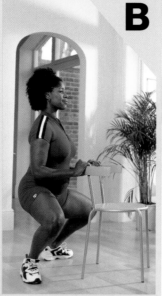

B

Bottom (gluteals)

2.Squat or plie

Stand facing the back of a chair, feet slightly wider than hip-width apart, feet parallel if doing a squat, or slightly turned out if doing a plie. Lightly hold the back of the chair for support. Contract abdominal muscles, bend your knees and slowly lower to a comfortable depth. Keep your knees over your toes and back straight. (do not take your bottom below your knees). Keep the chest lifted and shoulders relaxed.

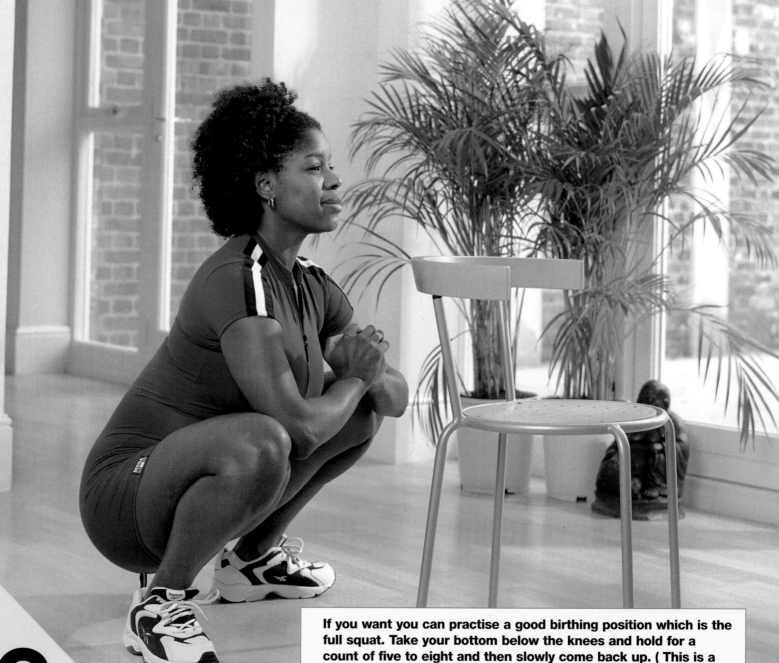

C

If you want you can practise a good birthing position which is the full squat. Take your bottom below the knees and hold for a count of five to eight and then slowly come back up. (This is a good position if your labour is slow as it tends to speed it up.)

Legs and bottom

1. Seated hamstring stretch

Sit on the floor with one leg straight out in front, knee soft, and the other leg bent to the side in a comfortable position. Place your arms on the floor behind you and tighten the tummy muscles. Press gently down on your hands and lengthen your spine. Keeping the arms on the floor for support, slowly incline your body forward until you feel a stretch in the back of the straight leg. Keep the knees and the toes of the straight leg facing up. Hold for the count of 10. Repeat with the other leg.

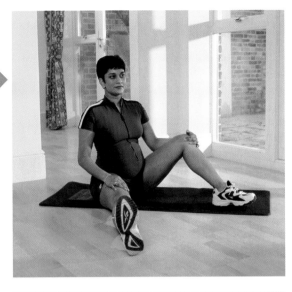

Legs

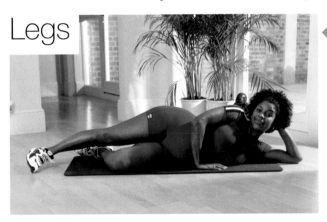

2. Side lying abduction

Lie on your left side with your head relaxed on your upper arm. Bend the bottom leg and straighten the top leg. Pelvic tilt and tighten the tummy muscles, roll the top leg forward so that the toes are facing the floor, and hip rotated forward. Slowly lift your leg slightly higher than hip height, and return to starting position with control. Change to other side. Do two sets of 15.

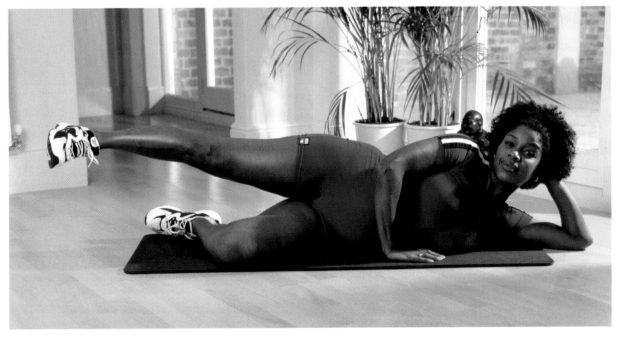

8

Breasts Chest

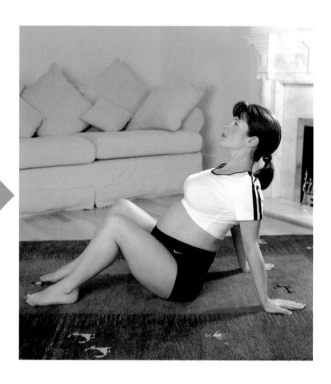

1. Seated chest stretch

Sit on the floor in a comfortable position, with your hands on the floor behind you. Tilt your pelvis, tighten the tummy and sit tall. Press down with the hands and lengthen the spine. Lift the chest and draw the elbows back, squeezing the shoulder blades together. Keep the tummy muscles pulled in to prevent the back from arching. Hold for a count of 30.

2. Chest press

Sit in an armchair slightly leaning back (being careful to prevent your tummy from 'doming' see Chapter 7). Hold a dumbbell in each hand at upper chest level, palms facing inwards. Tighten the tummy muscles and press up towards the ceiling. (Do not allow the elbow to lock out and keep the wrists in line.) Draw the arms down and back, keeping the elbows close to your body. Repeat 12 times.

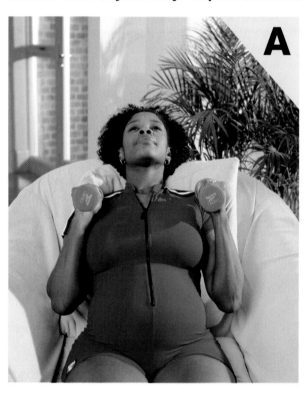

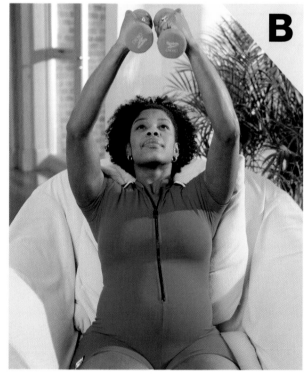

4. Repeat seated chest stretch

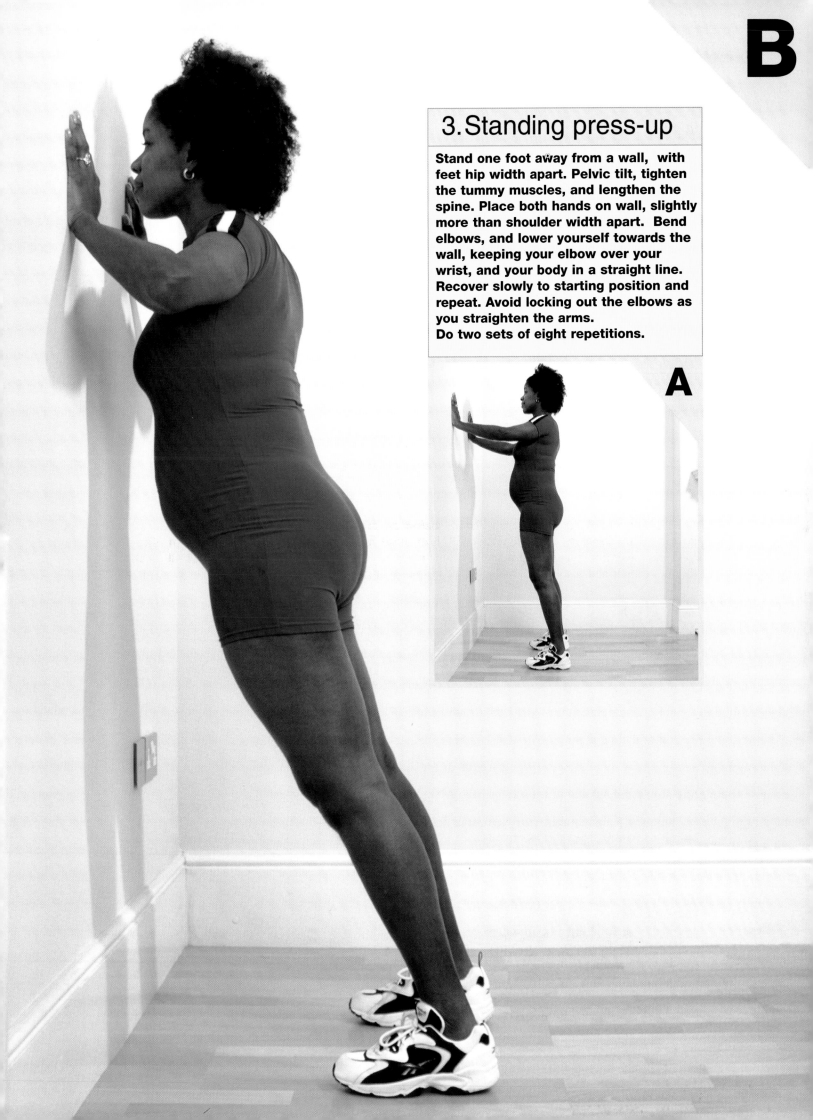

B

3. Standing press-up

Stand one foot away from a wall, with feet hip width apart. Pelvic tilt, tighten the tummy muscles, and lengthen the spine. Place both hands on wall, slightly more than shoulder width apart. Bend elbows, and lower yourself towards the wall, keeping your elbow over your wrist, and your body in a straight line. Recover slowly to starting position and repeat. Avoid locking out the elbows as you straighten the arms.
Do two sets of eight repetitions.

A

8

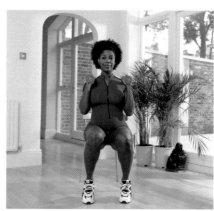

Shoulders and arms
Shoulders

1. Seated military press

Sit tall on the edge of a sturdy chair, knees bent and feet flat on the floor about hip width apart. Pelvic tilt and tighten your tummy muscles. Hold a dumbbell in each hand, with elbows bent and close to your sides. Forearms parallel and palms facing each other. Keeping tummy tight, slowly straighten your arms up and over head, taking care not to lean back. Avoid locking the elbow, and keep your hands apart, but elbows close to your head. Bend elbows and slowly return to starting position, keeping your elbows close to your side. Do two sets of 10.

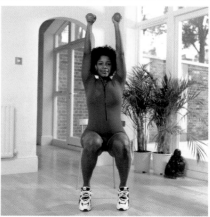

Cautionary note: if you feel light headed after raising your hands above your head, stop.

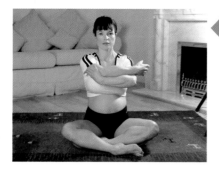

2. Upper back stretch

Sit tall on the edge of a sturdy chair, knees bent and feet flat on the floor about hip width apart. Or on the floor. Raise your arm up and across your chest. Support your arm just above the elbow with your other hand and gently ease it towards your body. Keep your shoulders relaxed, and the back lifted. Hold for 10-20 seconds. Repeat with other arm.

Arms Biceps

Biceps curls

Sit tall on the edge of a sturdy chair, knees bent and feet flat on the floor about hip width apart. Rest arms on your knees with a dumbbell in each hand palms facing towards knees, tighten your tummy muscles, and slowly curl the arm up towards the shoulder, rotating the forearm so the palms will face the your shoulder at the top. Keeping the elbows firmly into your side. Slowly return to the start position, taking care not to allow the elbows to lock out. Repeat eight times for two sets.

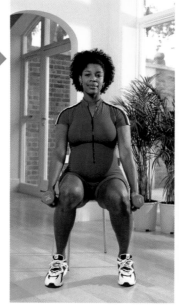
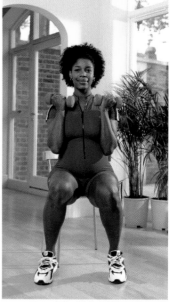

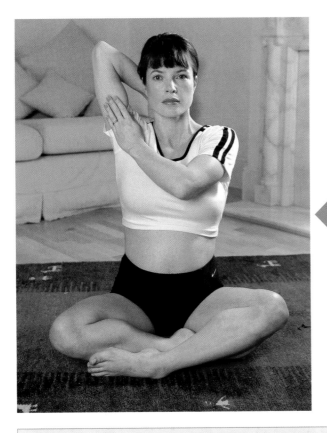

Arms Triceps

1. Seated triceps stretch

Sit tall on the edge of a sturdy chair, knees bent and feet flat on the floor about hip width apart. Or sit on the floor. Tilt your pelvis and keep the tummy tight. Lift one arm up to the ceiling, bend at elbow and rest arm between shoulder blades. With the other hand take hold of the elbow and gently ease behind the head; retighten the tummy muscles to prevent the back from arching. Hold the stretch for a count of eight. Change arms and repeat.

2. Bent over triceps extension

Leaning on the back of a high chair, rest one arm on the chair. Hold a dumbbell in the other. Feet shoulder width apart, legs bent and soft, pelvis tilted and tummy tight. Keeping the arm close to your side, lift the elbow up and back. Slowly extend the arm behind you, taking care not to lock out the elbow. Pause and slowly bend the elbow to lower the forearm. Keep the elbow lifted throughout and the palm facing inwards and wrist in line with the forearm. Change hands. Do two sets of eight.

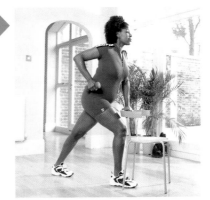

3. Repeat seated triceps stretch

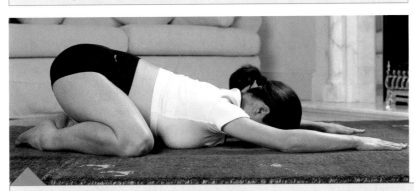

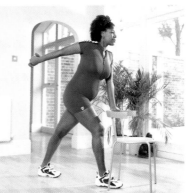

4. Bottom-up stretch

Kneel on the floor with legs as wide apart as is comfortable. Place hands in front of you and gently crawl forward so your arms are fully stretched out in front of you and your nose is close to the ground. You should feel the stretch all along your arms, back, your groin, and also in knees and ankles. Hold for a count of 10.

If you are suffering with varicose veins, this exercise can be done with the bottom up above the knees, taking care not to arch the back.

8

Pelvic floor

This is a hammock of muscles that support the bowel, bladder, and the womb. In pregnancy, the pelvic floor is able to stretch more in preparation for delivery. And this with the weight of the baby, creates extra stress. This can cause stress incontinence. You need to do pelvic floor exercises as often as possible. Done regularly this is another area where you can be stronger after pregnancy than before as we may not think of strengthening our pelvic floor muscles before we are pregnant.

You can be in any position, sitting, standing or lying – the legs should be slightly apart. Think about trying to draw up and close your back passage (anus) as if to stop yourself from passing wind. Draw up and close your front passage as if to stop the flow of urine. Squeeze and lift up inside the vagina. Remember to keep breathing rhythmical, hold for a few seconds then let go slowly. Try to increase the length of the hold up to 10 seconds. Repeat up to 10 times an hour. Do not hold your breath. Once you are comfortable with this technique, try doing some quick one second contractions as well as the long hold ones.

Relax in the recovery position

The front-lateral or recovery position is often the most comfortable when you are lying down. It may help to put a pillow under your upper knee. Allow a good space between your legs.

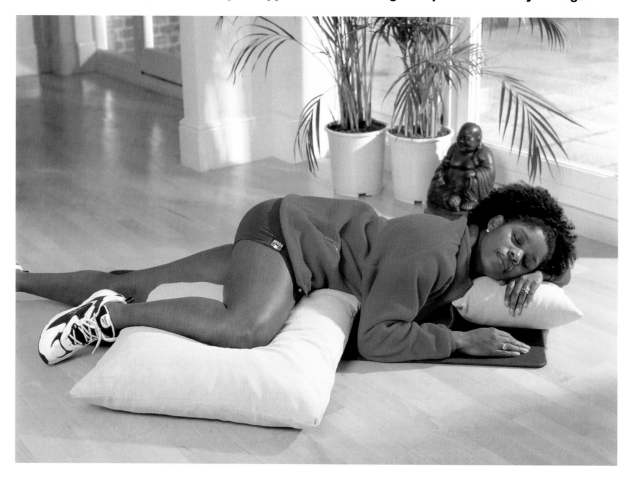

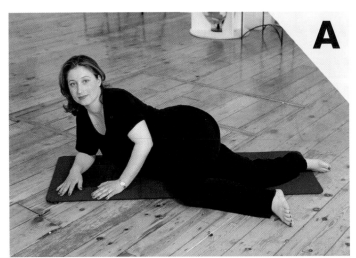

A

Getting up correctly

Whenever you are getting up from lying on your back, roll over on to one side first. Swing your shoulders round, and push with your upper arm, drawing up your knees at the same time, until you are in a kneeling position; tighten your buttocks and rise from this position. This movement is to avoid unnecessary strain on your abdominal muscles.

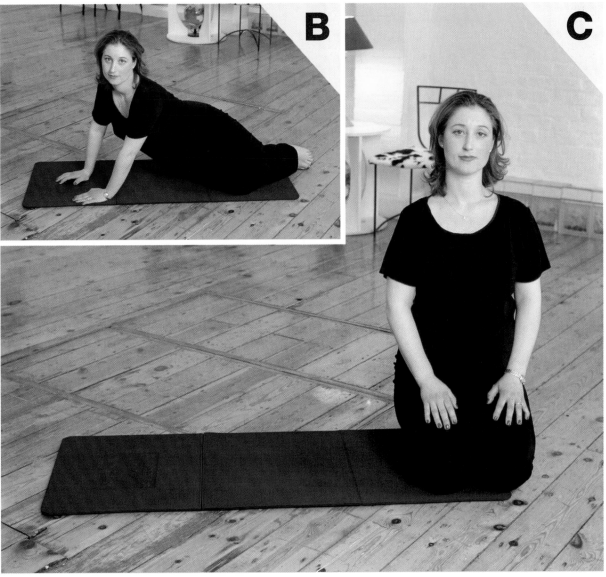

B

C

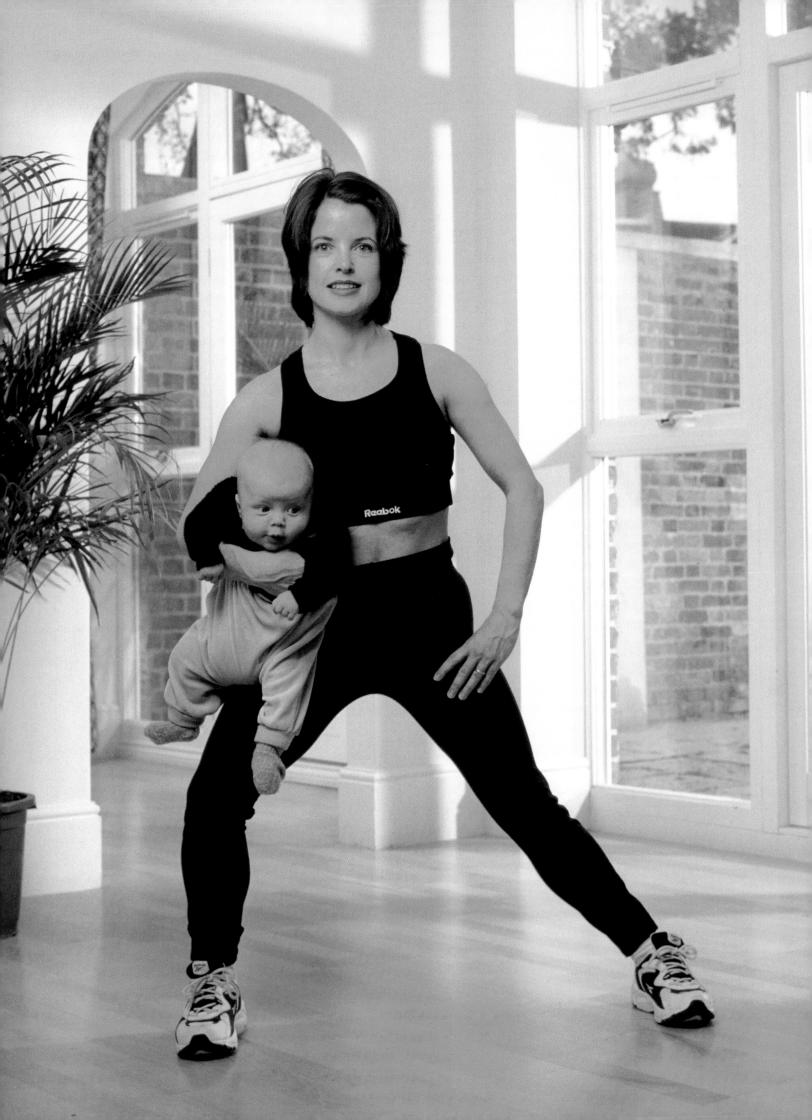

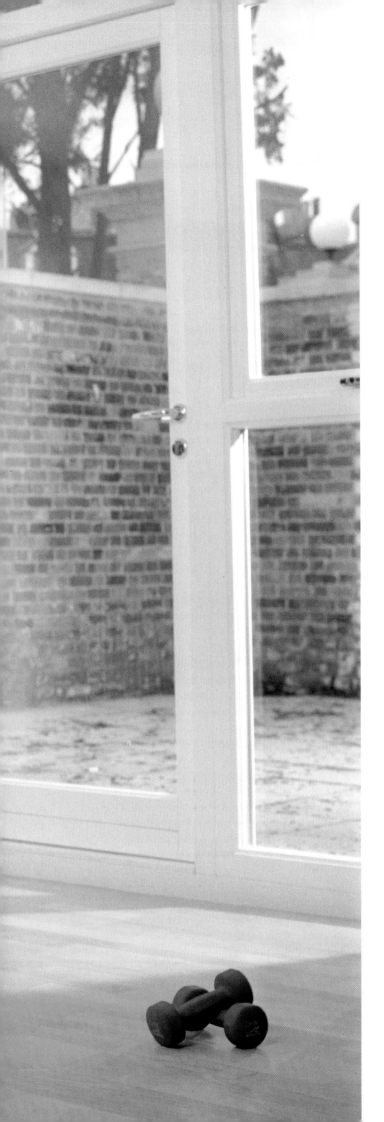

9

Exercises after Childbirth

E xercise is one of the most important components of postpartum recovery, but it is usually the last thing on any new mother's mind. There are some small, isometric (these are exercises that are of minimum movement but maximum tension) exercises that you can do soon after childbirth that will make a huge difference to your success at getting into shape.

When you start to exercise after you have had your baby, don't do too much too soon, no matter how fit you feel. Whatever your level of fitness, start with the simple, easy exercises we describe, and work your way up to higher levels of challenge as your body adapts to the previous level. Rushing too fast into an exercise routine that you're not ready for after childbirth will delay your getting back into shape.

Many women wait six weeks or longer after delivery before starting any exercise programme. For healthy women who delivered without complications, this is too long to wait. An immediate return to activity will optimise and increase these fitness gains, and will also start reducing the extra body fat. If you have had a difficult delivery or a caesarean section you may wish to check with your midwife or doctor before you start exercising.

Good nutrition especially if you are breast feeding is vital when following this, or any other exercise programme. Mothers who are well nourished will end up with the best results.

The first few days

The first 24 to 72 hours after delivery should be a time for rest, recovery, and relaxation. After a couple of days of complete rest, start with gentle walking, just around the house or, if you are still in hospital, around the ward. It is much more beneficial to be active than bedridden while you are recovering. If you have had a caesarean, ask for the okay from your doctor before you start walking. It is important that you start slowly, the emphasis is on rest, with some mobility, not the other way round. Being on your feet too much so soon after giving birth can cause fluid to build up in your feet (oedema).

Early walking helps to stimulate circulation, which in turn reduces oedema pain and stiffness. It encourages the digestive system, bladder and kidneys to return to normal functioning.

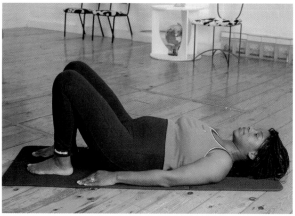
figure 1.

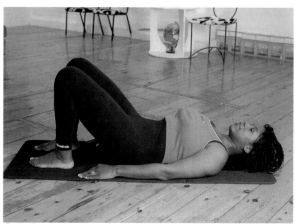
figure 2.

The first six weeks

Other exercises that will help you get back into optimal physical condition are pelvic floor exercises (see page 84) and abdominal and pelvic realignment exercises.

These exercises help you to:
● Regain proper alignment of the pelvic girdle
● Regain function of the abdominal and pelvic floor muscles
● Build a foundation from which you can work to maximise your physical state
● Prevent postural, and lower back problems which may result from weak abdominal muscles.
● Prevent poor urinary control, haemorrhoids, and prolapse of pelvic organs which may all result from weak pelvic floor muscles.
● Heighten sexual pleasure when strong.

It is also important to exercise these muscles because they will not regain tone naturally.

If you have had a vaginal delivery, with or without an episiotomy, the pelvic floor muscles will be extremely stretched and loose. Even with a caesarean section, they will be weakened.

Pelvic floor exercises
Pelvic floor (Kegel) exercises (see page 84) are very important after childbirth. Try and exercise your pelvic floor muscles as often as you can. The more you do, the more you will improve muscle tone in your stretched perineal area. You can do these exercises anywhere and, as you continue, you will notice these muscles getting stronger.

Abdominal exercises
As you start tightening your stretched abdominal muscles, they will feel very weak. You may not feel them at first, this is entirely natural as they have been stretched enormously during pregnancy. Doing the following exercises will help to shorten and strengthen your stretched abdominals:

Belly breathing
Lie on your back in bed, or on the floor (figure 1). Bend your knees, keeping your feet flat on the floor. Breathe in and expand your abdomen. Contract your muscles as tightly as you can, pulling your navel in towards your spine (figure 2). At the same time, tilt your pelvis upwards, bringing your hips towards your lower ribs. Make sure that you keep your bottom on the floor. Begin by doing as many as you can and build up to 15 a day.

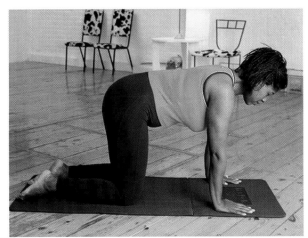

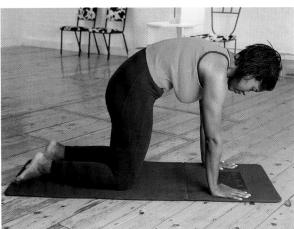

Tummy contractions and cat stretch (see page 87)
These are perhaps the most important of the realignment exercises. Do 4-6 of each of these exercises every day. They stretch your back muscles, which can be quite sore and also gently strengthen your tummy muscles. It may feel as though you have lost control of your tummy muscles, but stick with it and the feeling will return.

Hold your tummy in
Holding your tummy in re-establishes your abdominal posture, and reminds you to maintain correct posture in your back.

Walking – From delivery to six week check
This is just a general guide, remember to listen to your body and do what feels comfortable.

day	minutes of gentle walking	number of times a day
3	5	2-3
4	10	1
5	10	1
6	10	2
7	15	1
8	15	1
9	15	2

Exercises after six weeks

We all have a six week check because that is the time that the medical profession deems that our bodies have settled down physiologically. Though your body may not have returned to normal, you should be feeling a little more like your old self.

This is a good time to increase the duration of your walks, and combine this with some strength training. This combination is the most effective way to rid yourself of excess fat, and rediscover lean, toned muscles. Go through the 15 minute programme three times per week. (Or for a longer duration if you feel up to it.)

Try to match each strength training session with an aerobic conditioning exercise.

Tips when starting off
● Be organised. Set a particular time of the day for exercise
● Have a set place in the house which will be your 'place' for strength training
● Rather than fitting in exercise when the baby is sleeping, try to arrange a babysitter so you don't have the anxiety of hoping that baby doesn't wake up, and can concentrate fully on yourself (trying to avoid the frustration of baby waking when just starting to exercise)
● If you have stairs, put the changing table upstairs so you are frequently climbing those stairs each day
● Put on some music with an up tempo beat
● Monitor your progress by the mirror, tape measure, and bathroom scales (if you must) in that order
● If you're breast feeding, try to exercise when your breasts are not full, and wear a good supporting bra
● Team up with another new mother, exercise is often more effective when you have a person of similar ability to encourage you and keep you company
● Doing a little is better than nothing.

Aerobic conditioning

After childbirth, you should still be careful about high impact activities as relaxin will continue to make your joints more mobile for a few months after delivery. If you have exercised during pregnancy, your body will be fitter than before but may not be able to tolerate high impact exercises unless you allow it to gradually re-adapt.

Walking

Walking is one of the best fat burning exercise for postpartum women (see Chapter 3). You can get this valuable exercise as often as you like without the need of a babysitter.

Take your baby outside for a walk every day. It's good for both of you – your baby will nap better in the fresh air, and get fewer colds. Fresh air seems to toughen up the lining in the nose and lungs. Even if it is winter, try to get out for a walk. You and your baby will benefit. As well as losing fat, you will not be stuck in the house all day.

Breathe deeply as you walk. Check your posture and hold those abdominals in tight. Don't try to get your heart rate up. Just feel your circulation increasing. Progress to 10-15 minutes of walking, and use the 'talk test'.

Then walk for longer periods, working up to 30 minutes or longer. Remember that the more you walk, the more fat you will burn.

Resting heart rate

Take your resting heart rate by taking your pulse in the morning before you get out of bed. You should get a figure between 70 and 100 beats per minute (If you are very fit your pulse rate will be much lower.)

Your maximum heart rate is the number of beats per minute your heart can work at during peak exertion. It is extremely unsafe to work at maximum heart rate, during cardiovascular exercise you should aim to work at 70-80% of maximum heart rate. Halfway through your walk, you can work out the rate at which you are working. To work out your maximum heart rate you simply subtract your age from 220.

Warm up

Be sure to warm up. Walk at an easy pace for five minutes, then stop to stretch your calves.

Cool down

When you're coming to the end of your walk, slow down to warm up pace for at least five minutes. Then stretch your legs and hip flexors, holding each stretch for 20 to 30 seconds without bouncing.

Guide to walking - level one aim for

Week 1	15 minutes 3 x week
Week 2	15 minutes 4 x week
Week 3	20 minutes 4 x week
Week 4	20 minutes 5 x week

Guide to walking - level two and three aim for

Week 1	20 minutes 4 x week
Week 2	20 minutes 5 x week
Week 3	30 minutes 4 x week
Week 4	35 minutes 5 x week

Depending on how much more fat you wish to burn, you can either increase your walking times, up to an hour, or put in another day. If you have reached your ideal shape do at least 20 minutes three times a week to keep you fit and healthy.

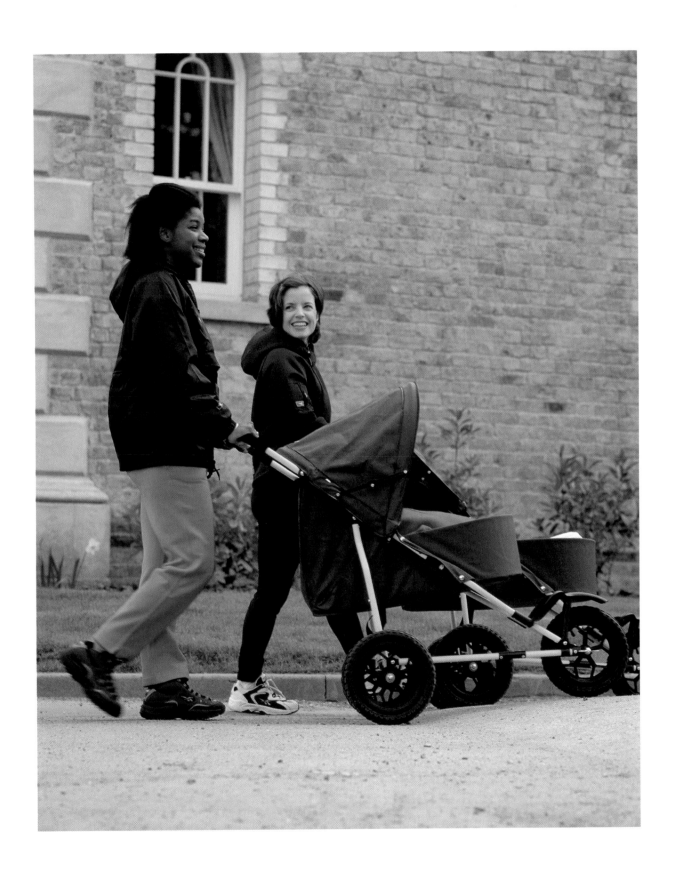

Strength training

Once you feel confident and comfortable with the aerobic programme you can add these exercises to your postnatal programme. The routine will take you 20 minutes. Aim to do it three times per week. If you are starting strength training for the first time, start off with 1kg dumbbells. If you have exercised with dumbbells before, start off with a lighter weight than you are used to and work back up to your usual weight. You can also use an exercise tube for some of these exercises. Remember that your joints are still unstable from the effects of relaxin for up to five months after delivery.

Warm up

1.Marching on the spot

March briskly on the spot, bending your elbows and gently swinging your arms forward and back. Lift your knees to a comfortable height, avoid letting the hips swing from side to side. Repeat for up to two minutes or until you feel quite warm.

3.Shoulder rotation

Stand with your feet slightly wider than your shoulders. with your arms relaxed and by your sides. Remember good posture. Slowly circle one shoulder back and round in a large exaggerated manner. Repeat five times on each side, then five times circling both shoulders.

2.Squat swings

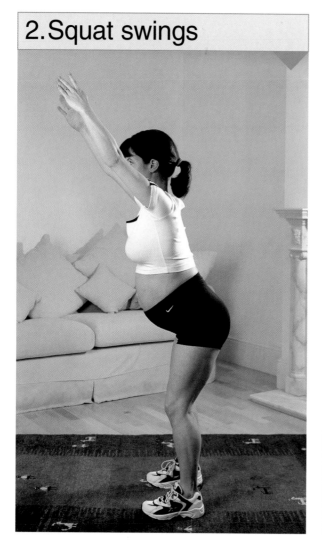

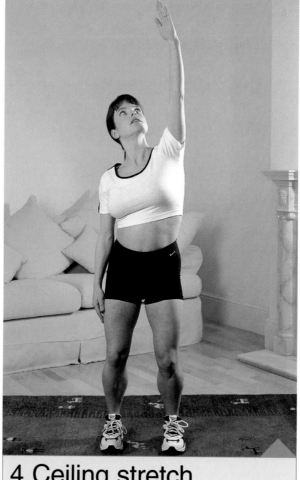

4.Ceiling stretch

9

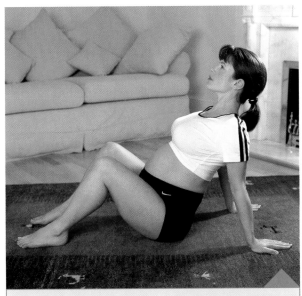

1. Seated chest stretch

Chest exercises

3. Pectorals

Sit upright with your knees bent and your feet flat on the floor about hip width apart. Tilt your pelvis and tighten your tummy muscles. Place your exercise tube around your upper back and under your arms. Hold the handles at chest level and press forward so that your arms straighten and your hands come together. Return slowly. Keep your wrists in line with each other and do not lock your elbows.(If you want to make this exercise more difficult, hold the tube below the handles.) Repeat for two sets of 12 repetions.

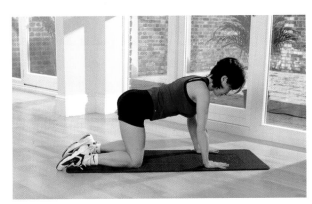

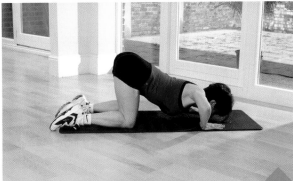

2. Press ups

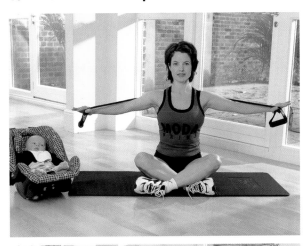

Kneel on your hands and knees, with your knees under your hips. Your hands should be slightly wider than your shoulders and your fingers facing forward. Bend your elbows and slowly lower your body towards the floor. Keep your head in line with your spine and your elbows over your wrists. Tighten your tummy muscles to keep your back from arching. Keep your weight forwards as you push slowly up to the starting position, taking care not to 'lock' your elbows. Repeat 8-10 times.

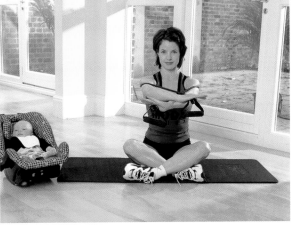

4. Seated chest stretch

Back and Shoulders

5. Upper back stretch

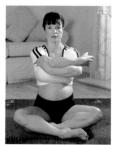

Sit tall on the edge of a sturdy chair, with your knees bent and your feet flat on the floor about hip width apart. Or sit on the floor. Raise one arm up and across your chest. Support your arm just above the elbow with your other hand and gently ease it towards your body. Relax your shoulders and lift your back. Hold for eight to ten seconds. Repeat with the other arm.

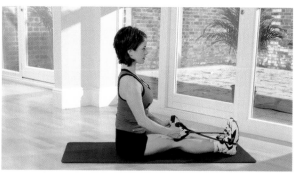

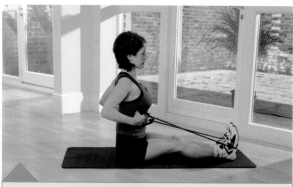

6. Seated rows

Sit tall on the floor with your legs out in front. Loop the tube around your feet and hold it firmly with your palms facing in, and your arms extended. Squeeze your shoulder blades and pull your arms back. Return to the starting position with control, keeping your tummy muscles tight. Do not lean backwards from the hips. Do two sets of 10 repetitions.

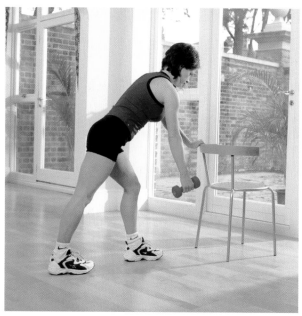

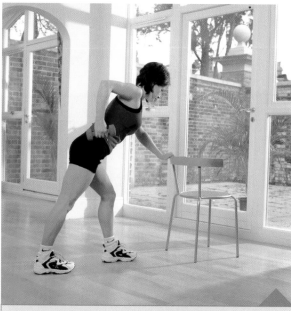

7. Single arm rows

Stand with one foot in front of the other with a wide base, and support yourself with one hand on the back of a high chair. *Posture check.* Hold a dumbbell in one hand and, in bent over position, fully extend the arm forward and down, but do not allow the elbow to lock. Keep the arm facing forward, and the wrist in line with the forearm, bring the elbow back so dumb bell reaches the waist. Repeat 12 times on each side.

8. Upper back squeeze

Sit cross-legged on the floor and hold your exercise tube in both hands, 10cm in from the handles on each side. For a greater resistance, put your hands closer together. Hold the tube at chest height, with your arms bent and your elbows lifted. Squeeze your shoulder blades back and together, pulling your elbows behind your back. Remember to breathe. Keep your tummy muscles tight to prevent your back from arching, and keep your shoulders down. Hold for a count of three, and gently release to starting position. Do two sets of 12.

9. Standing lateral raises

Stand with good posture, feet slightly wider than hips and knees soft, not locked. Rest your arms in front of your body with elbows slightly bent. Slowly take your arms out to the side and raise to just above shoulder level. Keep your shoulders down and the front of the weight facing down as though you are pouring out of a glass. Keep your tummy muscles tight and your spine lengthened throughout. Lower slowly to the starting position. Repeat for two sets of 12.

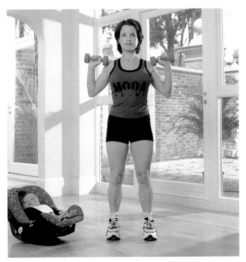

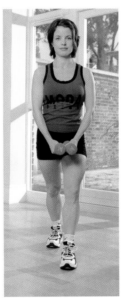

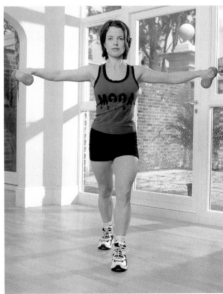

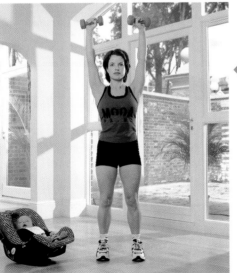

10. Military raises

Stand as with lateral raises. Hold a dumbbell in each hand with elbows bent and close to your side, forearms parallel and palms facing out. Keeping tummy tight, straighten your arms up and over your head, taking care not to lean back and avoid locking elbows. Keep elbows close to your head. Bend elbows and slowly return to starting position keeping elbows close to your side. Repeat for two sets of 10.

11. Repeat upper back stretch

Arm exercises

Bicep curls

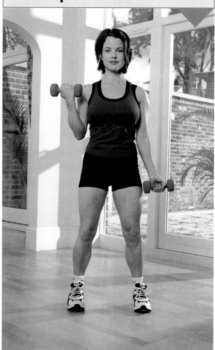

Do two sets of 12.

1.Triceps stretch

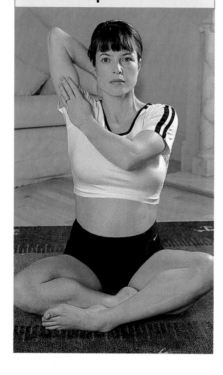

2.Dips

You can do these on a sturdy chair or a low bench. Place your hands on the edge of a chair and slide your bottom off the chair so that your arms are supporting your full body weight. Bend your elbows and drop your bottom towards the ground until your arms are bent at 90 degrees. Straighten your arms until you get back to the starting position. Repeat 8-10 times. If you want make this exercise more difficult, straighten your legs.

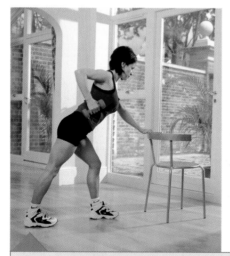

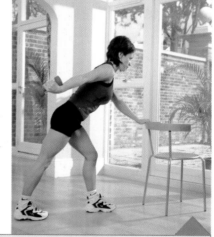

Do two sets of 10.

3.Bent over triceps extension

4.Stretch your triceps again

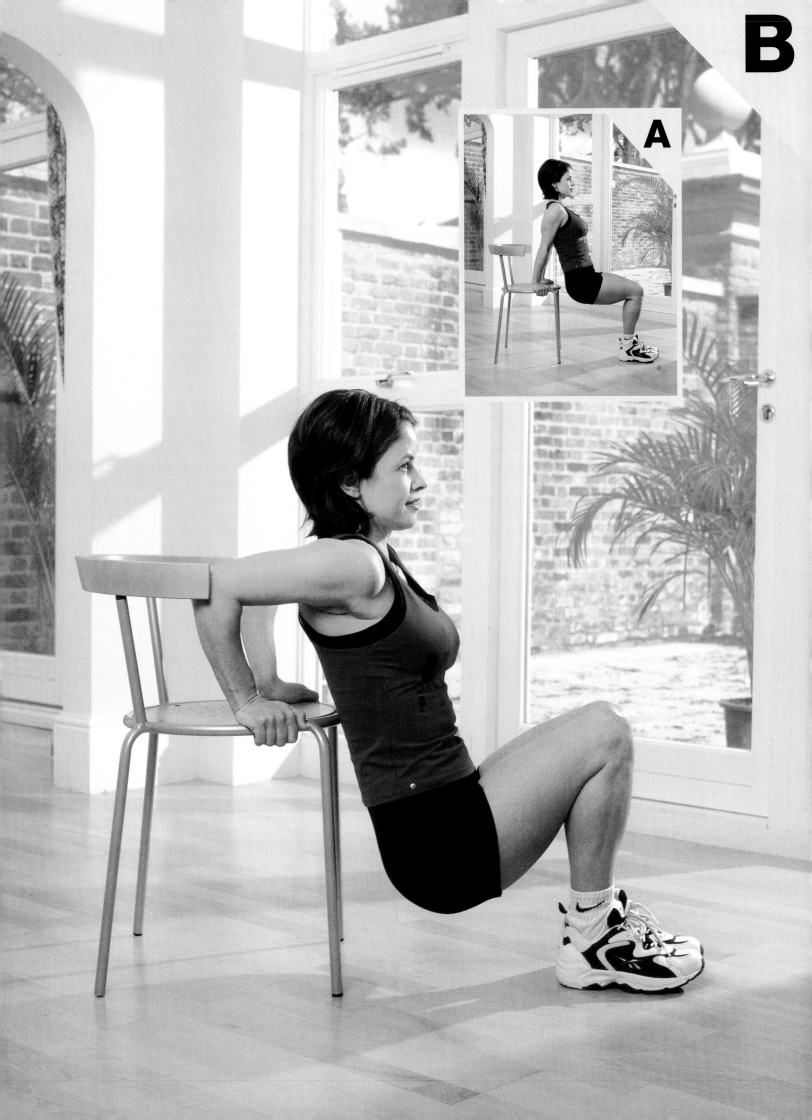

B

A

Bottom and thighs

1.Hamstring stretch

Sit on the floor with one leg straight out in front, knee soft, with other leg bent to the side in a comfortable position. Place your arms on the floor behind you and tighten your tummy muscles. Press gently down on your hands and lengthen your spine. Keeping your arms on the floor for support, slowly incline your body forward until you feel a stretch in the back of your straight leg. Keep the knees and the toes of the straight leg facing up. Hold for the count of 30. Repeat with the other leg.

2.Squats

Stand with your feet shoulder width apart and your hands by your side. Squat down till your thighs are parallel to the ground. Hold on to the back of a chair if you feel unstable. Look slightly above eye level to maintain a straight back. As you go down your knees travel in the direction of your feet and bring your arms forward for stability. As you push up, bear the weight on your heels. This should be a slow and controlled movement. Repeat 8-10 times or until your muscles feel sore.

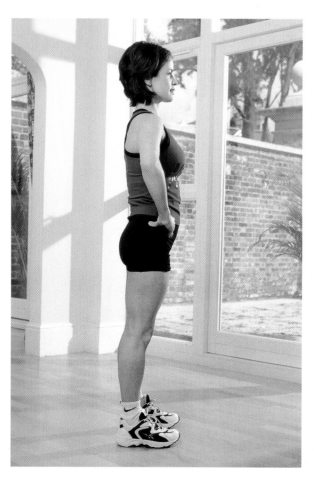
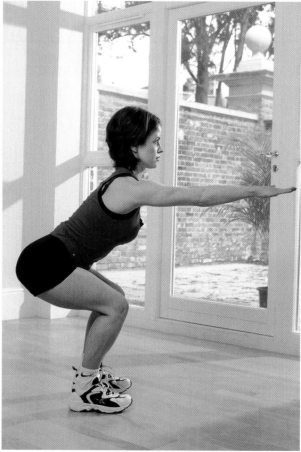

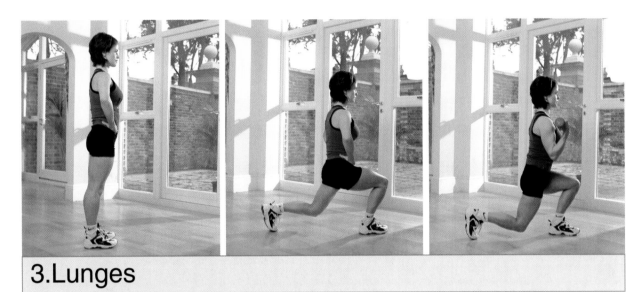

3.Lunges

Standing tall, step forward with one leg and lower your back knee towards the floor. Keep your front knee over your ankle. Keep your pelvis tilted, tummy muscles tight and back lifted throughout. Squeeze your buttocks tight and slowly return to the standing position. Repeat with the other leg. Repeat 10 times for each leg.
When you feel strong enough you can do this exercise with dumbbells for added resistance.

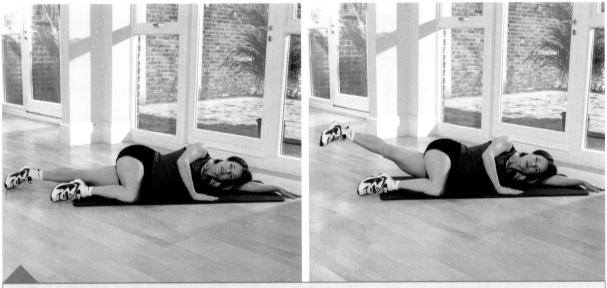

4.Inner thigh (adductor) lifts

Do not try this exercise if you have pain or discomfort around your pubic bone. Lie on your side with your body in a straight line. Place one hand under your head for support, the other in front of you to help stabilise your torso. Keep your bottom leg extended and bend your top leg over in front, so that your toe touches the floor. Tilt your pelvis and tighten your tummy muscles. Lift and lower your bottom leg. Focus on squeezing and controlling your inner thigh muscle. Repeat 20 times, then change sides. When you are strong enough, do another set.

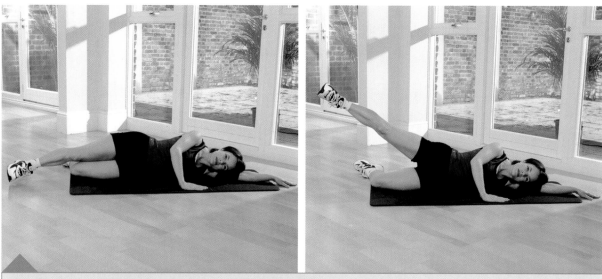

5.Outer thigh (abductor) lifts

Lie on your side with your head resting in your hand or arm. Bend your bottom leg, keeping your hip rotated forward and your pelvis tilted, tummy tight. Lift your top leg slowly up and down, keeping your toes just off the ground. Repeat 20 times, change sides. When you are feeling stronger do another set.

6.Repeat hamstring stretch

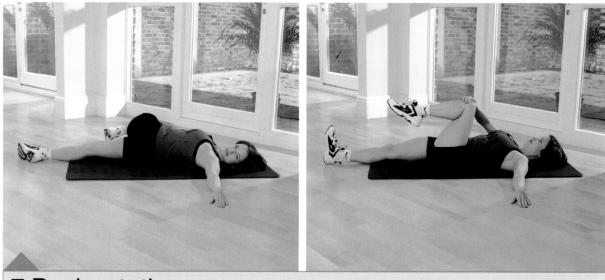

7.Back rotation

Lie flat on your back and extend your legs. Flex one knee and raise it to your chest. Grasp your knee or thigh with one hand. Breathe out and gently pull your knee across your body to the floor, keeping your elbows, head and shoulders flat. Hold the stretch for the count of 30 and relax. Repeat with the other leg.

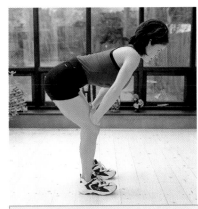 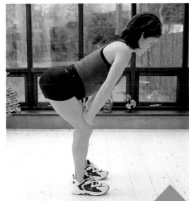

1. Standing stomach vacuum

First thing in the morning, before breakfast, slightly bend your knees, place a hand on each knee. Expel the air from your lungs and vacuum your stomach in, then release. Repeat three times working up to 10.

Abdominals

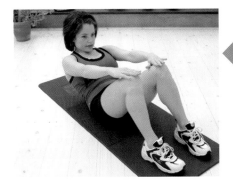

2. Basic crunch

Lie on your back with knees bent and shoulder width apart. Place hands gently on knees, fully extend arms. Tighten your tummy muscles, breathe out and slowly curl yourself up, keeping your tummy pulled in and flat. Pause, then slowly uncurl. Repeat 8-10 times.

3. Half curl sit ups

Start as above, but have your feet in the air knees bent at about a 90 degree angle. Place your hands by your ears (resting, do not pull your head). Focus your attention on your abs and squeeze so that you raise your shoulders off the ground, hold, then release and lower with tension.

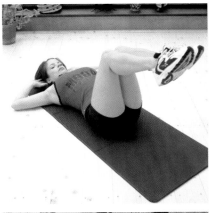

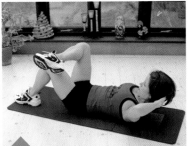 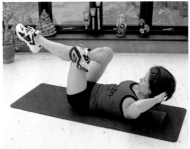

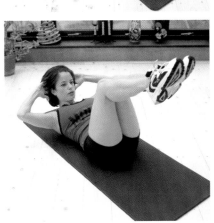

4. Single leg half raises

Lie on your back with knees bent, shoulder width apart. Bend right knee place left foot on right knee. Keep head on the ground. Lift right foot off the ground about 30cm then slowly return. Repeat 8-10 times or till your muscles feel sore.

10

Putting it all together

U p to now we have discussed effective ways to reshape your physical appearance after childbirth. In this chapter we look at the mind. The American philosopher William James said 'The greatest discovery of my generation is that human beings can alter their lives by altering their attitudes of mind'.

Here we will explore ways in which you can reorganise your life so that you have more control over its events and as a result have greater peace of mind.

Our roles in life

Women today are busier than we've ever been. Modern life means that we have to learn to juggle to survive. Many of us fulfil four major roles, which all use a great deal of our time, energy, and skills. We are:

● wives or partners
● mothers
● working women
● homemakers.

These secondary roles may also require our time and energy:

● daughter
● sister
● friend
● relation
● godparent.

Depending on your circumstances, these roles may be as significant as the primary roles or much less so. To cope with modern life, you have to learn to manage all these demands, as well as meeting other people's needs, to achieve balance. Many things conspire against you. They may be external factors, such as a baby who won't let you sleep, or a bullying boss; or internal factors such as low self-esteem and negative thinking. To cope successfully you need to adapt, change, or accept your circumstances to reduce stress. Coping successfully is vital in the postpartum period, and can set you up for true wellbeing long afterwards. Many coping strategies will allow you to fulfil your many roles and still feel good about yourself and other people, feel good about life itself, and embrace all the new

challenges that life will throw at you. For Tonia and me, the role which is not one of the primary roles, but supercedes all of them, is that of Christian. A love of God is at the centre of our beings, and is our foundation for the effectiveness of any coping strategy.

I don't want to preach religion to you. You could also say a love of goodness, a love of truth, a love of honour, integrity, joy, it's all the same. It's a pure, positive, universal energy that is greater than you.

You may think that some of the strategies we suggest overlap and repeat each other. We believe that the more you read these words, the more you will repeat them to yourself, the more will you do them. They will become long-term instinctive behaviour changes, instead of short-term concepts you quickly forget.

I suggest that you write things down. By doing this you make a visual commitment to yourself to aspire to goals and achieve them.

Stress is both a negative and positive factor. Negative stress (distress) zaps our energy and enthusiasm for life. It's the stuff that we're always trying to get rid of, reduce, and avoid. Positive stress (eustress) motivates and energises us to pursue relationships, engage in projects, and accomplish our goals.

Before you choose a method to combat stress, ask yourself where the stress comes from. If outside factors such as a new baby and relationship difficulties are causing stress, then a positive thinking or imagery-based technique may be effective. If the stress is based on the feeling of adrenaline in the body such as when you are working under pressure, it may be effective purely to relax your body and slow the flow of adrenaline.

Your partner

Your partner may be as stressed as you, but in different ways. He may feel that the weight of the world is now on his shoulders. Before they have babies, very few couples think ahead to a time when one of them (usually the mother) is no longer earning. It is a discussion couples find very hard to initiate. Money worries can cause a lot of anguish, and be compounded by tiredness and exhaustion. It is important that you talk about all these feelings and issues, so that they don't build up and lead to resentment and fights.

Our suggestions for fighting stress are directed at you, the new mother. But your partner can use many of the techniques to tackle stresses in his own life.

Positive coping strategies

Immediate remedies
Maintain a balance in life. Make time for work, friends, family, community, school activities, and religious activities. Always take time for yourself. Choose activities that nurture and pleasure you, like a hot bath with scented candles, fishing, flying a kite in the park, or doing nothing.

Laugh often. Laugh at the silliness around you, and try to see the funny side of serious situations.

Keep the BIG picture in mind. Getting upset over trivial or insignificant details adds nothing to your life. Ask yourself, 'In the big scheme of things, how important is this?'

Monitor your thoughts. What you think about affects how you perceive and interact with the world. Instead of 'I can't do anything about this,' use 'I'm going to give my best effort to figure this out' and there will be a positive outcome.

Relax daily. Give your mind and body a break. We give some advice on relaxing later in the chapter.

Successful stress management

There are many aspects of successful stress management:

● building self-esteem
● assertiveness
● goal setting
● positive thinking and positive affirmations
● empowerment
● organisation, time management, and the importance of routine
● physical appearance and body image
● visualisation
● exercise and nutritional habits
● relaxation

Self-esteem
It all begins with self. Your self-esteem, or how you think about yourself physically and mentally, is the most important ingredient of effective stress management not just postpartum, but in life generally. People with low self-esteem often have trouble dealing with negative situations, and deal with stress destructively. People with high self-esteem are positive people who feel good about themselves. They can turn a negative situation into a positive one in other words, they deal with stress constructively.

Low self-esteem can also affect the way you use other strategies for effective stress management. If you have low self-esteem you may also think negatively, feel disempowered, be reluctant to set goals for yourself, not exercise, and have a poor body image.

You are particularly susceptible to low self-esteem in the postpartum period. It may stem from feeling less in control of your life, and also from poor body image after the birth of your baby. Incorporating a fitness programme into your life, and starting to see your body get back into shape will give you higher self-esteem, and improve your postpartum adjustment.

To effectively manage stress, you must have high self-esteem. You must love and respect yourself. Our sense of worthiness tells us whether we like ourselves, and it affects our self-confidence and self-respect. If you think of yourself negatively, you will look at others negatively and not see good things in them. This can make you resentful, even bitter, and lead to envy and jealousy. It is destructive. If you look at yourself positively, you will view others positively, and see more joy and beauty in other things.

Have you also noticed that negativity is contagious? If you spend a lot of time around negative people, you will soon start thinking along the same way. I used to work with someone who always saw the negative side of life whether it was getting a piece of work completed or her relationship with the world. Eventually her husband left her, and she sank even greater into this pit of negativity and self-pity. She truly thought that she was the most unfortunate person on the planet. Though given much support, she never saw the positive side of anything. Spending time with her was mentally and physically draining. Eventually I tended to avoid her so that my positive attitude was not eroded.

Putting it All Together

Quality survey

If you have low self-esteem, change can only come from a willingness to face the truth. Honestly examine the reasons why you have low self-esteem. Write them down. Perhaps you feel that you haven't reached your potential personally and professionally, or you may feel that you are not doing yourself justice looks wise, and if you lost some fat and changed your hairstyle, you'd be quite stunning. Once you acknowledge these reasons, and understand why you have low self-esteem, you can go about changing it.

Next, write down positive things about yourself. For example 'I am a loving person', 'I am generous', 'I am honest', 'I am kind'. Also write down your physical attributes such as 'I have beautiful hair, I have a nice smile'. Then focus your energy on adding more things to the list, especially the qualities that come from within. When you are feeling down, look at that list to remind yourself of all the positives about yourself.

If you feel unsure about your mothering skills, add to your list 'I am a good mother and no-one can love my child like I do'. Having a baby changes you in so many ways, for some it totally empowers them because they have the destiny of another being in their hands, for others it can make them insecure because of the unknown now in your life. Say to yourself 'I can do this and I can do it well'. Keep repeating it. You are a mother now and the way you feel about yourself profoundly affects your child . You want these effects to be positive and loving, so love yourself, realise your own self worth and by doing this you are loving your baby more.

You are unique. There's nobody like you. Always remember that.

Assertiveness

Assertiveness is an important booster of self-esteem. Don't confuse it with aggression. Assertiveness means standing up for the things that you want and believe in while still respecting the wants and views of others. Aggression means using force to get what you want without considering the wants and views of others.

Being assertive means knowing what you want, and being prepared to use fair means to get it. You will listen to others, and if you feel that your way is right, will reason with them rather than forcing your way upon them.

Assertiveness is a quality that we should strive for. It earns respect, and gives you more self-respect knowing you are not willing to compromise your beliefs and values.

Being assertive also means that you tend to avoid confrontations, as people tend to think twice before provoking an assertive person. Mostly people who habitually provoke arguments tend to be bullies. Bullies are cowards, so will not cross an assertive person.

Assertiveness is vital for a new mother. Being assertive means that you can politely:

- ask for help when you need it
- tell friends and relations that you would rather that they didn't visit just yet, unless they are willing to get you a bit of shopping and maybe do some ironing
- tell your mother that you respect and value her views and of course she's done it four times before, but you would rather bath the baby your way
- make time for yourself ask your partner or someone that you trust to look after the baby for an hour or two so that you can relax, exercise, go for a massage, whatever makes you feel good

You will find that assertive people:

- are charming – they know that complimenting a person makes them more likeable
- are confident – they believe in what they say and do which makes them less likely to be shy.
- are not afraid of using 'I', implying ownership
- ask questions rather than taking things for granted
- can maintain eye contact when they are talking to you
- are not afraid to say NO.

Goal setting

Setting goals will also enhance self-esteem and make you more disciplined. Setting and achieving goals can define success, but do not label yourself a failure if you fail to achieve them. Fear of failure often stops us from challenging ourselves by setting goals. Develop a little empathy and understanding for yourself, then relax and enjoy the journey.

You'll see that potential roadblocks become minor detours on your way to developing the body that you want, and a healthy outlook on life. If you are afraid, you won't go anywhere. You'll just hide inside your own self-inflicted wall of fear. Don't let excuses or fear dominate your actions.

Tips for setting goals

Goals should be specific, measurable, achievable, realistic, and time limited. No-one else need see your goals unless you want them to, be honest with yourself

Try setting some short-term goals that can be achieved in a week or a month. At first, choose things that you are pretty sure you can accomplish.

When you achieve a goal, even a small one, take time to acknowledge it to yourself, give yourself a pat on the back, and feel the positive energy.

Then try to extend your goals. The further the range the more expansive your imagination can be, so that your horizons are constantly extended.

If you do not achieve a goal, do not criticise yourself or assume you have failed. Simply note that this did not happen and decide why. If you want to set it as a goal again first work out why it did not happen the first time. Then write it down, imagine it already achieved and it will come.

Don't take on too much at once. Set goals that feel good to you. If you feel out of control, overwhelmed and insecure, try to simplify your goals. The whole point to this is to make your life more enjoyable, so find goals that make you feel this way.

Positive thinking

To think positively is vital for self-esteem. Writer Iyanla Vanzant says that 'you become what you believe, and get what you expect'. If you think negatively, negativity will come into your life.

The postpartum period is a time when you are very susceptible to negative thinking and feelings. Fatigue and hormonal changes mean that you have to work hard to banish negative thoughts from your mind.

Don't say 'I just can't cope', or 'I'll never again have a flat tummy', because if you think negative thoughts, negativity is what will manifest itself into reality. You won't cope, and you won't lose your tummy.

Believe in yourself. If you do, others will too, and you can achieve whatever you set out to do. Say 'I can lose the fat', 'I can handle whatever life throws at me'. Say 'I can' and you will. Before you shut your eyes each night, think about all the good in your life, about how fortunate you are, about how great it will feel to take control over your life.

Be grateful for what you already have, and grateful for what you have the ability to achieve.

People like to hang around positive energetic people. You become like the sun, with other people circling around you like planets, living off your positive mental attitude.

Positive affirmations

Positive affirmations are vital for high self-esteem, and needed by everyone. If you have a supportive partner, family or friends, they will constantly build you up with positive affirmations such as 'you're a great mother', or 'you're a special, loving person'. Particularly in a partner, some of the more silent types may not say these things, but will show them in other ways.

If you do not get positive affirmations from others you can get them internally by telling yourself, and believing them. Giving yourself positive affirmations is more valuable than hearing them from other people. It will foster self-belief and self-confidence, and reinforce your feelings of worth. When you tell yourself these things, you will believe them, and people around you will believe them too.

I use positive affirmations like these:
- I have a kind heart
- I acknowledge my faults and try to be the best that I can be
- I will always do right by my child
- I strive to be a beautiful person, and inner beauty will manifest itself externally.

Both Tonia and I also constantly give positive affirmations to our children, and make a conscious effort to avoid the negatives. Though they are just toddlers, we are constantly telling them that they are clever, special, kind, generous, beautiful inside and outside. It will install these beliefs in their minds, and make them believe those things in themselves as they grow up.

Being positive will instil values in them that will guide them through life.

Empowerment and working life

Empowerment is a source, or feeling of control that comes from deep within. Being in control gives you a sense of power. If you feel unempowered, you will feel that external forces control you.

Being empowered will make you feel not only that you are in control of your life, but that you have the power to change your life. This is an important part of stress reduction. The arrival of a new baby is frequently a time for focus and clarity

Putting it All Together

10

about your life, and the life you want for your baby. As well as the huge love you will feel (either straight away or a bit later), you and your partner will also feel an overwhelming sense of responsibility. Suddenly you have this little being to provide for, and you may decide that you have to make drastic changes in your professional life to provide a glorious future for all of you and subsequent others.

High self-esteem, setting and achieving goals, being fit and healthy, being happy with your body image, loving yourself, all add up to a feeling of empowerment. Being empowered means that you become your own boss. I mean that figuratively, but I would also like to mention mothers in the workplace. Many women find that having a baby leads them on to different career paths as they realise that being a 100% mother, and a full-time worker are incompatible. A survey of 5000 working women conducted by a women's magazine and the medical group BUPA, found that 77% of career women would give up their jobs tomorrow if money were no object. Many said that they were underpaid, overworked, and under such pressure juggling the roles of mother, homemaker, and full-time worker, that it was damaging their health. The average age of the women was 36, and 84% of them said that they believe women perform too many roles nowadays. This is backed up by Canadian study which found that career women who raise a family face a greater risk of stress-related illness than their husbands. While tensions at work raise the blood pressure of both sexes during the day, working mothers remain stressed far longer into the evening and night, increasing the dangers of heart disease and stroke. In contrast, men find it easier to switch off and relax at the end of the day, allowing their blood pressure to return to normal within a couple of hours.

Many women who choose to stay at home as full-time mothers are also under a great deal of pressure. It can also be very isolating spending all day with a young child or children when all around you are going to work and having adult conversations. Going out to work gives a little distance from your children, which in turn makes you miss them.

More and more women are today choosing self-employment, working from home, or attempting to start their own businesses after starting a family. Advances in communications, such as e-mail, make this much easier than ever before. Though working for yourself has its own stresses, the stress you create for yourself is possibly more bearable than stress created by your employment, over which you have no control.

Self-employment means that you have more control over your working hours, and lessens the strain of trying to fit childcare into a traditional working day. But it is a big step, which must be carefully thought out and planned.

After the birth of my daughter, I was working for a large news agency, which I found boring, uninspiring, and required no creativity from me. Dr Christianne Northrup, in her book *Women's Bodies, Women's Wisdom*, states that blocked creativity can make you sick. I believe this to be true. I resigned soon after returning from maternity leave not entirely sure what I wanted to do. I had made a list of what I wanted from life, and what I had to offer knowing that I wanted to use my creative energy to make a difference in the world. (See page 138)

I have found that being self-employed requires the five S's. They are:

- **Self-discipline** to make sure that you use your time constructively and are not easily distracted
- **Self-confidence** to go out and promote your business and talk to potential customers, potential partners, bank managers, etc
- **Stamina** to be able to put a great deal of your energy into your project, while still having the energy to keep the home and take care of your family
- **Sacrifices**, as you may have less money initially, you will have to go without certain things such as new clothes and eating out for a while. You may also see less of your family and friends. But tell yourself that it is a temporary measure for a glorious future and you won't mind too much
- **Slog**. You will need to put in a lot of work when starting up, and work very long hours.

Real success is being in a job that you love.

Organisation and time management

You know the feeling that you get when you have a good clearout of old clothes and ornaments, and take sackfuls to the local charity shop? As you rid your wardrobe and rooms around the house of clutter, you immediately feel lighter as if you've also got rid of clutter from your head. We carry far too much information around in our heads, and it causes clutter in just the same way as overcrowded rooms.

Being organised, managing your time, and setting a routine are important skills for managing stress. I always carry a notebook wherever I go. In it, I make lists, and sub-lists of my lists. Phone-calls, shopping, or a television programme to watch, they all go on my list. That way my mind doesn't have to carry around that information, so I have less 'mind clutter'. I prioritise my lists, so that if I don't get through everything, I at least get the more urgent things done. Crossing things done off the list, however small, gives me a great sense of achievement.

There is plenty of anecdotal evidence that brain activity is affected by pregnancy and childbirth. Many of us feel that our brains turn to mush, especially in the first few postpartum months. What is probably true is that because a new baby requires so much of your time and focus, you are unable to devote your attentions to other things. So becoming a new mother is the ideal time to get into the habit of successful organisation, good time management, and routines.

Even with a new baby, you can adopt routines that help your baby to feel totally secure. Your child will grow up more disciplined, and more able to spend time by himself. When we cope well with stress, we are also teaching our children to handle it well.

How to organise your time
Make lists of everything you need to do, or remember throughout the day

Learn to delegate. Most family members can help with baby related chores. You don't have to do everything yourself

Decide when in the day you are at your best, so you can be most productive then. Rest when you know you are at your least productive.

Prioritise, and get the most difficult things out of the way first.

If you are constantly procrastinating over something, decide whether you really want to do it, then set a time to get it done.

If you can, hire a mother's help, or just a cleaner to help you a few days a week during the postpartum period. If you can't, make arrangements for a mother, sister, or friend to help.

Set aside a time for household chores. Try doing them when the baby is awake, either strapped to you in a carrier, or in a rocker. That way you can rest when he sleeps.

Set aside a time for you, when you can exercise, have a facial, or read. The most organised and clutter-free house in the world will not make you happy if you are unhappy with your appearance.

Tonia writes: If you are not very organised, and trying to get organised is causing more stress in your life than the chaos you live in, relax and don't worry. I did not have a routine after I had my first child; we just seemed to float along. I spent a lot of time with my extended family, and bedtimes would vary. This way of being suited my situation, and I was happy; if I had tried to set a more rigid routine at that time it would not have suited my lifestyle. However, this easy going way could not continue once my child became older and I had another. We have at least a good 'going to bed routine' and that keeps me sane, because no matter how hectic the day has been 'bath, milk and story' settles the children and gives me the evening!

How to manage stress as your baby gets older
Make meal time family time. At breakfast, sit down with your child or children for at least five minutes. Ask about their plans for the day and what they are looking forward to. Tell them about your plans. It starts the day on the right note.

Schedule family fun and fitness time. Do something active anything, as long as it's together.

Streamline your life. Do you, and your child, really need to do everything you are doing? Re-examine your priorities. Simplify. Make sure you have energy for what's important. At bedtime, spend at least 10 minutes relaxing with your child. Let your child chat about what he or she wants. See the world through your child's eyes. Read a story together. Nobody's perfect and everybody makes mistakes. Before you go to sleep at night, think about one thing that you did well that day.

When you do feel stress, try to recognise it and deal with it. Relax. Take a deep breath. Try to figure out exactly what is bothering you. Sometimes your attitude can make the situation more stressful than it really is.

Talk with someone about your concerns and worries. Take care of yourself. Get enough rest and eat well. Take some time for yourself.

Positive body image
Positive body image is vital to high self-esteem and successful stress management. How you see and feel your body, and how others view it determine your body image. It is your most tangible aspect. We live in a society where physical beauty gets you ahead, and most of us strive for it. We feel more confident when we are looking attractive, than when we are unkempt and scruffy.

Putting it All Together

10

Improving your body image through fitness, leads to higher self-esteem, greater self-confidence, empowerment, physical and mental strength, self-respect, independence, and trust in your own decisions. Everyone can take positive steps to improve their body image through exercise and good nutrition.

Tonia writes:

'Why was it that only after I had a baby that I finally have the body I had wanted? It was because I had finally allowed myself to have a good body image instead of a bad one. During my pregnancy it was acceptable to have a belly so I relaxed and enjoyed the changing of my shape. I was able to eat well for my baby, and exercise for her too. I let go of all my self-consuming negative thoughts because there was someone else to consider. My life suddenly came clearly into perspective, my priorities changed and my body was not the first thought on my mind, my baby was. After I gave birth I held on to that positive image, I saw it in my mind's eye, over and over again till I finally became it.'

Visualisation

Visualising is a major key to stress management and success. It is a mental training technique which involves picturing a particular result. This gives you a mental blueprint that remains in your subconscious and subtly drives you toward your established goals.

Visualise how you want to look. If you are losing body fat, picture your physique as toned, slim, sexy, and curvaceous. As you train, you can constantly close your eyes and recall this mental image. You use your mind's eye to go over how your stomach will look eventually. You then programme your nervous system to respond to the programmed images in your head.

Visualisation builds confidence because it programmes your brain positively. It can block out creeping negativity by giving you something to focus on. If you do it regularly, you'll find a new link between your mind and body. Your concentration will increase, as will your confidence.

This exercise below will help you learn how to focus on the present. By paying attention to what is happening now, you increase your awareness and ability to create your future. Don't worry if it seems hard at first it will get easier each time you do it.

Focusing on the uniqueness of each moment is a powerful acceptance strategy. By accepting what is happening, we can imagine what we want to create in life and take action.

How to visualise

Find a quiet place away from distractions. I always use the 'peace' chair. This is an armchair in the living room, conveniently placed next to the fish tank, which is only to be sat on when you want peace and relaxation.

- Get into a comfortable position and relax your body.
- Take a number of slow, deep breaths.
- Release tension, concerns, and anxieties as you breathe out.
- Imagine that your mind is a TV or computer screen.
- Clear the screen.
- Imagine the number one on your mind's screen. Focus your attention on it. Allow other thoughts and feelings to go away.
- Allow the number one to fade and begin to visualise what you want to achieve. Imagine each figure, the scenery, the setting, filling your picture with the minutest details. Add vivid colours to your picture. Make the colours bright and dramatic. My place resembles Teletubbyland.
- When your picture is complete, add the sounds that are associated with your picture. You might hear yourself saying words, others talking, birds singing, or waves crashing.
- When the volume is turned up, fill your picture with the smells and tastes that are associated with it, such as the fragrance of flowers, the ocean air.
- Add the sensation of touch. What does the picture feel like in the sense of textures and temperature?
- Enjoy the full picture you've created.
- Add the critical element to your visualisation your emotions. It's the emotional element that expertly transfers your picture into your brain's memory cells. With your picture in full array, add to it the emotions you want to feel when you find yourself in this situation. Whatever the emotions pride, sorrow, joy, confidence, patience, gratitude, love – feel them fully. Allow your body to respond to the feelings associated with your pic ture. Smile, beam, gesture, what ever way you express your emotions. Hold your feelings in concert with your picture. Fully be in the picture you've created for yourself.
- Once you've held your picture strongly on your mind's screen for a few minutes, let it fade gradually until you return to your focus symbol the number one.

Exercise and good nutrition

Taking exercise and eating well are so beneficial to postpartum recovery physically and mentally. Physically they improve your body image at a time when you can be unhappy about the way you look, and mentally because exercise eases tension, and the better you look, the better you feel. Mind and body are inextricably linked. You cannot fully develop your mind without stretching your body.

Relaxation

Relaxation is an important stress manager. Regular spells of deep breathing, relaxation and meditation reduce stress hormones and strengthen your body's immune system. When your mind is relaxed, you can help to heal the damage caused by stress, and recharge your batteries. When you relax, you're escaping from the every day bombardment of stimulation and demands. You restore your energies, reduce the clutter in your mind, and can maintain a sense of peace about your self and life.

Everyone can use a daily dose of peace and relaxation, but it is especially beneficial for an expectant or new mother to make a habit of relaxing. Regular relaxation can counteract the stresses of your daily activities.
The basis for all mind-body relaxation techniques is to let go. You don't have to worry about doing it right. Put aside your daily concerns for a few moments. You can return to them after your session. The idea is to relax, really relax. There are many relaxation techniques. Common to all is the purpose to 'be' with yourself and not 'do'. In 'doing' our focus shifts from relaxing to achieving. While hobbies, such as reading and gardening, are relaxing because they're different from the work we do, in the pure sense of 'being', they don't count. Ways that do count include:

● gentle stretching
● massage
● listening to sounds and music
● visualisation
● breathing awareness
● meditation.

If you can combine these in a weekly routine you can start to redirect your energies into more creative and productive channels. You may feel deep physical relaxation and a greater sense of inner wellbeing.

We believe that relaxation is essential to daily living. When you can relax regularly you can improve your health and boost the quality of your life.

How to relax

Find a quiet, comfortable place where you won't be disturbed.
● Sit or recline in a comfortable position, with your whole body, including your head, supported
● Don't worry about a 'right' way to relax.
● Set a time limit for yourself, and gradually work up to

30-45 minutes as you become more comfortable with the technique.
● If you want to make a change in your life consider what that change is. Briefly make a picture of it in your mind then let it go. Changes happen more easily when we are in a relaxed state.
● Fix your eyes on one spot.
● Focus on your breathing, allowing yourself to breathe fully and freely.
● If you need to, move your body to get really comfortable.
● Make statements to yourself of whatever you are aware of seeing, hearing, or feeling.
● Make three statements of things you see, three of things you feel, and three of things you hear. Then make two statements of each, then one statement of each. And then close your eyes. With your eyes closed repeat the cycle of 3-2-1 statements of what you see, hear, and feel.

Allow your body to rest and your mind to wander as if in a dream. If your goal is simply to relax, you may imagine a very peaceful scene or remember a pleasant experience. If you have set a goal for yourself to make a change, you may imagine times in your past when you had the resources that you need for change. See yourself in the future having all the skills and resources that you need to accomplish your goal. When you are ready to come back to your fully conscious state, once again make statements of what you are aware of.

When you have finished, keep your eyes closed and just sit quietly and without effort for two to three minutes. Allow yourself to come out of the relaxation gradually before opening your eyes and resuming your activities. You will feel awake and refreshed, as if after a good night's rest.

Relax daily and when you're feeling out of balance or frustrated. Even two or three minutes can be helpful.

Keep trying, even if you find it difficult to relax at first. When you relax, you escape from the everyday bombardment of stimulation and demands. You restore your energies and reduce the clutter in your mind. The systems in your body are given an opportunity to slow down and work more efficiently. You increase your enjoyment of life, you can focus on what's truly important, and you can maintain a sense of peace about your self and life.

Because relaxation is something we do for ourselves, it's usually the last thing we think about, our concern is generally taking care of others first. But we do a much better job of helping others meet their needs when we're conscientious about meeting our own, including relaxing and nurturing our bodies.

Putting it All Together

10

Stretching

Stretching helps reduce tension in the body's muscles. You can use the stretches we recommended for use before and after your aerobic or weight workout. But do them deliberately and twice as slowly as usual. Breathe deeply during the stretching. Breathe in to begin the stretch and slowly breathe out as you complete it.

Massage

Massage has its origins in the athletic and medical practices of Greece, Rome, and ancient Chinese medicine. It can be beneficial in dealing with chronic neck and shoulder tension, and is increasingly being used during or after pregnancy for its positive relaxing and health enhancing effects. Being massaged by another person is a great way to 'be' while tension in the muscles and toxins in the body are released. There are various massage techniques, including sports, deep tissue, neuromuscular, Swedish, and Oriental.

You may have to try out a few massage therapists before finding one that uses a technique that suits you. Ask friends for recommendations and ask the therapist to show you their certificates of accreditation.

Listening to music

Listening to certain types of music is a great way to relax. Classical music is very relaxing, but the type of music to choose is subjective. Nature music such as bird sounds and whale noises are believed to enhance creativity. Instead of listening to talk shows or the news on the radio, play music that will relax your mind and body and nurture your spirit.

Visualisation

Visualisation can take you on a trip for little effort and without any expense. To relax through visualisation, close your eyes and create a relaxing scene with your mind's eye.

Breathing awareness

Breathing is the simplest and perhaps one of the most effective relaxation techniques. You can use it anywhere to relax. Without breath, life doesn't exist. Breathing is the foundation for all relaxation techniques. The deeper you breathe, the deeper you relax.

Using breathing to relax

- Begin by breathing deeply and evenly
- Fill your lungs and your abdomen with air
- Release the breath slowly through your nose to a slow, deliberate count of five. As you breathe out, release the tension and worries that have built up
- Continue to breathe in and out for at least five minutes.

Progressive relaxation

When you relax progressively, you tighten and release each part of the body by itself on both sides. Begin either with your head and move down, or your feet and move up. To begin with your lower body, firmly tense your toes as tightly as possible and hold the tension. Then, very slowly, release the toes. Now, move up to your feet. Firmly tense them, hold the tension, then slowly release the feet. Continue the tensing and releasing until you reach the top of your head. You can tense and relax both sides simultaneously or one at a time.

Autogenic relaxation

This is similar to progressive relaxation in that you involve the whole body one part at a time. Rather than tensing the muscles, you'll say, 'My toes are warm' three times and feel the blood moving to that part of the body to warm it. Then you move to the feet. 'My feet are warm.' You'll find that your muscles are more relaxed when they're warm.

Nature

Being in nature is a lovely way to relax. Listening to the movement of the wind and water and to the sounds of the animals and birds is enjoyable and refreshing. Fresh air invigorates the body's cells. Find a park you can visit during lunch time or on your way home from work to release the day's worries.

Yoga

There are many types of yoga, including Hatha, Kripala, Iyengar and Kundalini. Hatha is perhaps the most relaxing of them all, the postures are stretches that are held for an extended time and are co-ordinated with the breath. Yoga classes are often taught in community and adult education centres, health centres, and yoga centres. Ask your friends for recommendations.

Meditation

There are also many types of meditation including Transcendental Meditation (TM), Primordial Sound Meditation, Kundalini Meditation, complete silence, and mindfulness meditation. Many forms of meditation require a teacher, and again you could ask your friends for recommendations.

How to meditate by yourself

- Close your eyes.
- Breathe normally and naturally, and gently notice your breathing. Don't try to control or alter it in any way.
- Notice how your breath changes by itself. It may vary in speed, rhythm, or depth, and there may even be occasions when your breath seems to stop for a time.

● Whatever happens with your breathing, observe it with out trying to change it.

● Focus on your breathing for the whole time. For maximum benefit, do this for 15 minutes.

Try them!

If you can relax regularly, you will soon reap the benefits of mental clarity, a calmer disposition, less tension, and a more efficient body. Try all the techniques and find the ones that work for you. If you don't take time out to relax, you shortchange yourself physically, emotionally, mentally, and spiritually. There are many things in life you can delegate, but nobody else can relax for you.

Body Maintenance
Staying Motivated

Once you make up your mind to start the strength training and fat burning programme, or even once you have achieved your desired body shape, you will need to keep motivated. That way, you are more likely to continue exercising and eating healthily without it seeming like you are having to make a conscientious effort.

Tips on staying motivated:

● Do not start with too much too soon. If you are new to exercise, don't over-train or over do it. You will be in danger of giving up completely or injuring yourself.

● Schedule your workouts, and treat them as if you would any other appointment.

● Morning workouts are a good idea as you would have got it out of the way, and you start the day feeling that you've already accomplished something positive for yourself. However, later workouts also have their advantages.

● Eat only when you're hungry. Refrain from eating because others want you to, it's time, it's there, or you paid for it. Don't give in to pressure to have one more piece or just one more bite. If you eat because you're upset, make a list of alternative actions you can take in the place of eating when you're not really hungry.

● Concentrate on finding personal measures of improvement. Are you feeling better, or looking better, or losing inches around your waist? Any improvement will encourage you to continue. Remember to stay off the scales.

● Muscle weighs more than fat. If you must, weigh your self only once a month.

● When you feel like doing nothing, do a little. Many programmes are abandoned because the hour workout seems like too much and you end up doing nothing. On days like this, change your goal to 15, 10 or even 5

minutes, but just do something. Consistently doing a 5 minutes of strength training is better than doing 20 minutes rarely.

● If you're getting bored, change your workout. You could join a gym if you're getting bored of your workouts at home, or change your walk route.

● Make it fun. Train with a good friend. Train to music. Just try to make workouts fun, and not forced.

Just a little note to partners, to always give positive encouragement, NEVER use negative language like 'come on fatty', even in jest. These comments hurt and set negative images. If you really want to help your partner tell her you love her as she is. If she has some shaping to do, she will feel secure while she is doing it. If she feels secure she will be happy, if she is happy, you will also have a happier life!

Taking your eating and exercise plan further

Once you have stopped breast feeding you may now want to take your routine further. You are already on the road to a great shape by using the triple combination worked out in this book, now you may wish to sculpt your body a little bit further.

Now is the time to try to increase the weights you are using because when you strength train, you build up your muscle, and when you have more muscle, you burn more fat.

If at all possible the best times to do your aerobic exercises are when your stomach is empty, so even 5 or 10 minutes before breakfast get your metabolism going and taps into fat cells as your body's glycogen stores are low after a full night's sleep.

Also a couple of hours after your evening meal is a good time to go for a walk. An advantage of waiting until after dinner before taking a walk is that you may burn 50% more calories than if you wait to eat after you get back.

Try to eat the bulk of your carbohydrates early in the day, so have a good, slow burning carbohydrate breakfast, and lunch. If you have not done any exercise that day, try to restrict carbohydrates in your evening meal (stir-frying is a delicious way of eating like this and you do not even miss the carbohydrates).

This way, your body manages to use up all its glycogen stores and will tap into the fat stores. Do not eat late at night as it makes it harder for your body to metabolise food, so it is more likely to turn into fat, also you are more likely to over-eat if you save your main meal till late at night.

10

Bust maintenance

In Chapter 7 we talked about regaining a flat tummy after children. Apart from the tummy, another part of your body that shows the effects of pregnancy, especially if you breast fed your baby, are your breasts.

There's no denying that pregnancy and breast feeding leave a lasting impression on your breasts. They may, if you're lucky change for the better, but more than likely your breasts end up smaller and emptier once you've stopped breast feeding, or just as a result of pregnancy. As women get older, breasts change. You never quite get the full, convex look that you had in your teens, and for most, surgery or implants seem to be the only answer.

But that's not entirely the case. There are natural alternatives to improve your bosom, and though there is no scientific study that proves it, there is plenty of anecdotal evidence to suggest that you can increase the tone, and even size of your breasts by alternative methods.

The most effective treatments involve supplements containing plant derived oestrogens.

Other ways to improve your bust involve vitamin and mineral supplements, aromatherapy massage, hydrotherapy, creams and gels, and exercise.

Natural supplements

Trials carried out in a leading Sunday newspaper and a popular daily newspaper, on various methods of increasing the size of the bust, showed that a natural supplement called Erdic could actually firm and enlarge the breasts. To understand why Erdic works, we need to understand about the make-up of our breasts.

Each breast is made up of a gland surrounded by fat, and it is this fat that gives the breast its volume. After puberty, the amount of glandular tissue in the breast gradually decreases and is not replaced unless there is a surge of hormones in the body that causes the breasts to swell, such as during pregnancy and breast feeding. Erdic works because it contains plant derived oestrogen – phyto-oestrogen – from ingredients such as hops, buckwheat, oats, malt, barley, rye, wheat and corn.

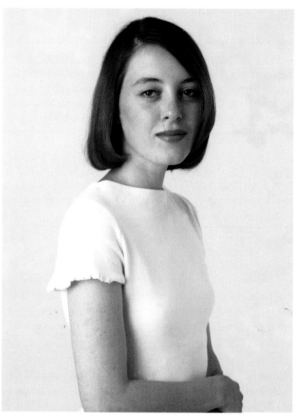

Lucy Marlow before her treatment with Erdic.

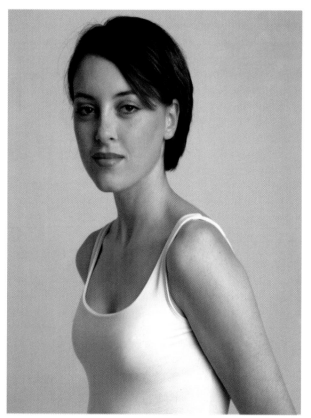

Lucy after.

The addition of phyto-oestrogen to the body stimulates the glands in the breasts to grow fatty tissue, hence the increase in size. It also increases the amount of glandular tissue produced, which provides the breasts with extra support.

Though excess oestrogen in the body can have potentially harmful side-effects and even promote the growth of breast cancers, phyto-oestrogen seems to mimic the body's oestrogen without having its harmful effects. Many scientific studies point to the health benefits of phyto-oestrogen in reducing breast cancer and the symptoms of the menopause.

Though there have been no clinical trials, there is plenty of anecdotal evidence to suggest that Erdic works:
Lucy Marlow found that her bust was smaller after breast feeding, but after taking Erdic for 10 weeks, her bust increased from 32A to 32B. Jo Cross also found that her bust increased from 32B to 32D after taking Erdic for 15 weeks. American nutritionist Ann-Louise Gittleman has also taken Erdic with positive results.

Agnus castus is a herb which increases progesterone production, which makes breasts swell. It also boosts the

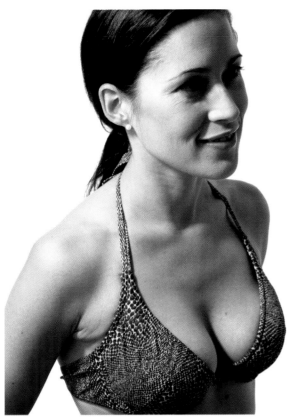

Jo Cross gained two cup sizes after treatment with Erdic.

production of prolactin, the hormone produced during pregnancy that stimulates breast tissue.Other plant derived oestrogens include red clover, wild yam, and black cohosh.

Vitamin and mineral supplements
Evening Primrose Oil and vitamin E help to strengthen the skin, improve elasticity and make the breasts look firmer. Silica, calcium flouride, MSM, vitamin B6 and pantothenic acid also help to strengthen the skin, and so firm the bust.

Aromatherapy massage
Oils such as grapeseed, rose, geranium, fennel, and clary sage are slight oestrogen stimulants so massaging them in a clockwise direction into the breast may boost firmness. Try 30ml of grapeseed oil, with three drops of rose and geranium, five drops of clary sage and four drops of fennel.

Hydrotherapy
Hydrotherapy works by massaging the breasts with cold water, which has a tissue firming effect. The concentrated water massage helps to firm the tissues, improve the elasticity of the epidermis, and avoid premature slackening of the skin.

Clarins Model Bust is a hydrotherapy breast massage that can be used at home to improve the bust

Creams and gels
Regular massage with an ordinary moisturiser will help stimulate circulation, which will improve the tone of the breasts.

Clarins have a range of bust gels, lotions and tonics, which contain some key ingredients for a healthy bust. They include ginseng, sage and witchhazel that tone and tighten, echinacea and ginkgo biloba that have a firming effect on the skin, and marine algae that strengthens the skin.

Gatineu's bust firming gel contains echinacea, tensine to tighten, and horsetail to firm.

Exercise
The breasts have no muscular means of support but 'sit' on the pectoral muscles, so having well toned pectoral muscles will help support the breasts and improve their shape.

Remember that it is important to always wear a good fitting bra, especially when exercising, as it will help slow down the impact of gravity.

10

Spirit

A mother is a mother still,
The holiest thing alive.
Samuel Taylor Coleridge

Earlier in the book, we have endeavoured to impart the best knowledge to maximise your potential physically and mentally. I felt that we had to add this part because of the profound way that having a baby changes not just your life, but you yourself. When you become a mother, you will not be the same being that you were before.

Even if after following the programme in this book you get back to looking the same, or better than before you were pregnant, you are not the same afterwards. You are deeply different on a psychological, social and spiritual level. You are a mother. You have created another human being who you are responsible for. Here I want to focus on those spiritual changes that motherhood brings about.

Spirit means different things to different people. I can define it best by saying that the creation of this book came from Spirit. It came from a power deep within, it guided me, and every word came from this same power. It is also called intuition, and my great lesson was to learn to trust this intuition, realise that it is connected to the greater power of the universe, and also listen for the messages that provided the guidance.

In other words, Spirit is about every thought we have, every word we speak, every deed we undertake. If you can connect with Spirit, you can draw on and benefit from the great power of the universe. And once you make this connection, you find a joy in all things living, a joy that helps you reconnect to nature. Your life will be richer and happier as you feel this connection to other life-forms, and with that joy comes peace of mind.

The connection of all this to motherhood is love.

Often a person comes to his or her spiritual side through failure or loss, whether it be the loss of a job, or the breakdown of a relationship. The pure unconditional love and undying compassion that a mother feels for her child can also lead you to your Spirit.

I once heard Spirit defined as growing love inside yourself. Pregnancy is the physical embodiment of that definition. This love grows for nine months, and though it doesn't seem possible, the love continues to grow as you nurture and care for your child, who will always be a part of you.

And when you become a mother, you become a mother to not just your child, but to all children, everywhere. You will feel pain when you read about or hear of a child suffering. And you will die before you will let anyone harm your child.

Engaging the spirit has little to do with religion. It has much more to do with recognising that we are all human embodiments of the energy that created us, and that we are all connected within the universe. Spiritual matters include learning about and honouring ourselves and each other, recognising that we all have access to the power of love, listening to and following our inner guidance, seeking truth, and living in the present moment.

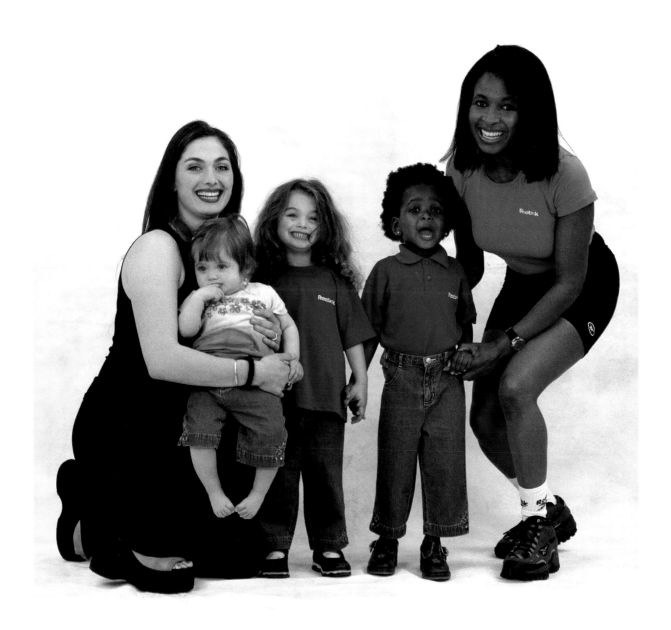

Index

Alternative holistic maintenance

Holistic healing is taken from the Greek word 'Holos' and it means treating the whole person, the body, mind and spirit.

We have listed some alternative methods of healing or preventing problems that can arise both during and after pregnancy; these methods can also help your baby if he is suffering from any ailments. These methods treat all of you, the whole person rather than a specific symptom. Just because many alternative methods are gentle and non-intrusive does not mean they are not very powerful at healing . Some treatments will suit you more than others, and all of them can work along more orthodox medicine.

Osteopathy

Osteopathy is concerned with restoring and maintaining balance in the neuro-musculoskeletal systems of the body. It is a complete system of medicine, using only manipulative and adjustive techniques to restore the body's self-healing power. It is a non-intrusive treatment, which gently corrects any imbalance in the body. Time and time again osteopaths see their subtle manual re-balancing techniques rewarded where more intrusive methods have failed.

The Osteopathic Centre for Children (OCC), is a fund run charity which is committed to the wellbeing of children and pregnant and postpartum mothers. Their long-term ambition is to have paediatric osteopaths as part of the obstetrics team and to attend the delivery room to check over newborn babies and their mothers. Although it is accepted as normal nine out of ten children suffer trauma in the birth process, only a handful of them is currently treated.

Chiropractic

Chiropractic works on the principle that the nervous system controls every part of the body, through the nerves that branch off the spinal cord from between each spinal joint. If the joints are not moving properly (as a result of poor posture, stress, accident or other factors) the nerves can be affected and cause discomfort, pain or even disease. Chiropractors relieve pain by manipulating (or adjusting) the joints and surrounding ligaments and muscles with their hands. They do not prescribe drugs, a fact that makes chiropractic an ideal treatment for pregnant women.

Studies show that 50% of women suffer with low back pain during pregnancy. In addition, instability of the pelvis and changes in posture may result in pain and discomfort in the pubic area, buttocks, groin, legs and other places. Chiropractors use a variety of techniques that are specially tailored to suit pregnant women.

Many mothers return to their chiropractors for a check-up after the birth of their baby, to ensure that labour has not led to further nerve irritation. Since birth is one of the greatest physical traumas most of us will experience, chiropractors advise that the baby is also examined and treated if necessary. Small adjustments early on can make a huge difference to a child's health later. The practitioner will gently adjust a baby's spine to remove nerve stress. A study in Denmark revealed that when spinal adjustments were given to 316 infants with colic, 94% of them were relieved of symptoms within a two week period of treatment.*

Reiki

Reiki is the Japanese word meaning Universal Life Energy, an energy that is all around us. It is possible to heal at any level of being: physical, mental, emotional or spiritual. The method of receiving a Reiki treatment from a practitioner is a very simple process. The recipient simply lies on a couch and relaxes. If they are unable to lie down the treatment can be given in a sitting position, the main thing is for the recipient to be as comfortable as possible. There is no need to remove any clothing as Reiki will pass through anything. The practitioner gently places their hands non-intrusively in a sequence of positions which cover the whole body. There is no belief system attached to Reiki so anyone can receive or learn to give a Reiki treatment, the only prerequisite is the desire to be healed.

Reflexology

Reflexology is a natural healing science based on applying pressure to minute points in the feet thereby creating a stimulating effect throughout the whole body. In an indirect way it works through the nerve pathways thus creating an energising effect from the tips of the toes through the nervous system culminating in the brain. Reflexology relaxes the body, mind and spirit, improves circulation and normalises bodily function. It can help with some of the symptoms of pregnancy and is extremely helpful in aiding body functions, like the muscle tone of the bowel, to prevent constipation.

Babies seem to love reflexology even while in the womb; most mothers say that as they have the treatment they can feel lots of fetal movement.

It is recommended that you continue to have reflexology right up to and including the early stages of labour. It also can aid recovery in the post-natal period.
The Egyptians used this science in 2500BC; certain Indian and African tribes believed in the healing potential of the feet; and today it is a very revived and beneficial therapy.

Bach Flower remedies

There are 38 Bach Flower remedies, each one dealing with a particular emotional state or aspect of personality. The remedies work on the mental/ spiritual level, so they do not interfere with modern medicine. Up to six or seven remedies can be given at one time, depending on need. It is important when diagnosing to take in the person's personality as well as mood in order to treat the whole person. The remedies are preserved in brandy, so it is recommended that they are diluted in water. The Bach Flower remedies can easily be self prescribed but if you have any queries you can call Judy Howard at the Bach Centre and they will give you advice (see page 144).

Mimulus – for fear of pain, childbirth or something going wrong

Mustard – for unexplained depression

Olive – for fatigue and exhaustion

Impatiens – for impatience and irritation to help relax in the last days and weeks

Rescue Remedy – to help the mind remain calm and in control and to ease pain and shock. (I always carry a bottle of rescue remedy around with me, if I feel myself getting tense I breathe deeply and take a couple of drops.)

Red Chestnut – for over anxiety

Star of Bethlehem – for shock due to traumatic birth

Elm – for feeling overwhelmed by the responsibility of parenthood

Homeopathy

Homeopathy is an effective and scientific method of healing which assists the natural tendency of the body to heal itself. It recognises that all symptoms of ill health are expressions of disharmony within the whole person and that it is the patient that needs treatment not the disease.

Hippocrates realised that there were two ways of treating ill health, the way of the opposite and the way of the similar. For example, when treating insomnia, the way of the opposite is to treat this by giving a drug to bring an artificial sleep. This frequently involves the use of large or regular doses of drugs which can cause side-effects or addiction. The ways of the similar, the homeopathic way, is to give the patient a minute dose of the substance which in large doses causes sleeplessness in a healthy person.

Surprisingly this will enable the patient to sleep naturally. Because of the minute dosage no side-effects or addiction will result.

Homeopathy is very subjective – what works for one person may not for another if the emotions, are different. It is very important to go and see a professional homeopath the remedies in this book are for guidance and can be used safely.

When taking a homeopathic cure avoid camphor, coffee, eucalyptus, menthol and peppermint (for example Vicks or Olbas.)

Aromatherapy

The word aromatherapy means treatment using scents, and that is exactly what it is. Aromatherapy is a treatment that reaches the very core of our senses through touch and smell, using the scents from aromatic oils to heal and uplift the body and spirit and to make us feel better mentally and physically.

Proper use of the oils helps promote a more balanced lifestyle. There is less likelihood to succumbing to everyday illness and the effects of stress.

A balanced state of mind promotes vitality and a better ability to cope with potentially difficult events, like coping with a newborn baby. Use of aromatherapy oils can also stimulate the immune system, avoiding that run-down feeling that can cause stress and unhappiness.

> **NEVER APPLY ESSENTIAL OILS DIRECTLY ON TO THE SKIN AND NEVER USE THEM INTERNALLY.**

References

*Klougart N., Nilsson N. & Jacobsen J. (1989) Infantile Colic Treated by Chiropractors: A Prospective Study of 316 Cases. *J Manip Physiol Ther*, 12 : 281-88

Appendix 2

Useful contacts

The Council for Complimentary and Alternative Medicine
206 Latimer Road, London W10
Tel: 0181 735 0632

Aromatherapy
School of Holistic Aromatherapy
108B Haverstock Hill, London NW3 2BD
Tel: 0171 284 1315

Bach Flower Remedies
The Dr. Edward Bach Centre
Mount Vernon, Sotwell, Wallingford,
Oxon. OX10 0PZ
Tel: 01491 834678
Fax: 01491 825022

Chiropractic
British Chiropractic Association
Blagrave House,17 Blagrave Street,
Reading, Berkshire RG1 1QB
Tel: 0118 950 5950
Fax: 0118 958 8946

Homeopathic Medicine
David B.Needleman
Cory Pharmacy
166 High Road, East Finchley
London N2 9AS
Tel: 0181 444 9966/7464
Fax: 0181 883 7578

The Homeopathic Helpline
09065 343404
calls charged at £1.50 per min.
open from 9am to 12 midnight 7 days a week

Massage Training Institute
24 Highbury Grove, London N5
Tel: 0171 2226 5313

The School of Meditation
158 Holland Park Avenue, London W11
Tel: 0171 603 6116

Organic Food. *Box schemes and home delivery*
Organics Direct
1/7 Willow Street, London EC2A 4BH
Tel: 0171 729 2828 / Fax: 0171 613 5800

Organics To Go
PO Box 17464, London E8 3UG
Tel: 0800 458 2524 (freephone)
Fax: 0800 458 2524 (freephone)

Osteopathy
General Osteopathic Council
Osteopathy House
176 Tower Bridge Road
London SE1 3LU
Tel: 0171 357 6655 / Fax: 0171 357 0011

Osteopathic Centre For Children
109 Harley Street, London W1N 1DG
Tel: 0171 486 6160

Personal Trainers
Association of Personal Trainers
Suite 2, 8 Bedford Court
London WC2E 9LV
Tel: 020 7836 1102 or 07970 971125

Reflexology
The British School of Reflexology
Holistic Healing Centre, 92 Sheering Road
Old Harrow, Essex CM17 0JW
Tel: 01279 429060 / Fax: 01279 445234

Reiki
The Reiki Association
Cornbrook Bridge House
Cornbrook, Clee Hill,
Ludlow, Shropshire SY8 3QQ
Tel & Fax: 01584 891197

Erdic
12 Harley Street, London W1N 1AA
Tel: 0845 604 0274/ www.erdic.co.uk

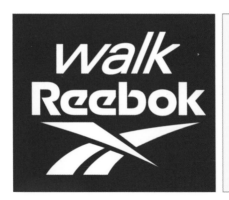

We outlined the many benefits of walking as a form of exercise in Chapter 3, however, getting started on a walking programme can be the hardest part.

Walk Reebok is a fitness programme which has been designed to turn walking into a workout. It adds specific movements to improve the aerobic benefits of walking, focussing on posture and technique.

Walk Reebok classes are available throughout the country. To find out if there is a *Walk Reebok* instructor in your area call 0113 237 1100.

Your child deserves the best
We'll help you provide it

At Milupa we're dedicated to providing information, advice and support to help you make an informed choice about your child's nutrition and development.

Join our **FREE** programme and we'll send you regular packs designed to give you the information you need at important stages of your child's growth, together with loads of **free samples** and money off coupons. Just complete the coupon below or phone **0845 601 0204** quoting MBK

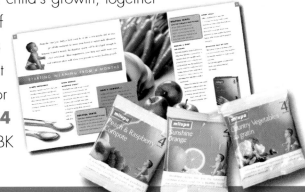

Cut out the coupon below and return it to:
MILUPA, FREEPOST NEA 2629, NEWCASTLE UPON TYNE NE12 9AA
No stamp required

- -

Title (MRS, MISS, MS, OTHER) _____ **Name** _____

Address _____

_____

Postcode _____ **Telephone** _____

Is this your first pregnancy? ☐ Yes ☐ No (please tick)

Date your baby is due _____

Are you expecting: **Twins** or ☐ **Triplets** (please tick)

Please send me information about the range of Milupa infant meals and milks (please tick)

Signature _____

I understand that I will be sent regular information by Milupa on their range of babyfeeding products.
Milupa reserve the right to modify the programme without notice. Please allow 28 days for receipt of first pack.
Please tick this box if you do not wish to receive offers from companies other than Milupa. ☐

MBK

milupa

Acknowledgements

We give thanks to God for His guidance in the completing of this book.

Special thanks to:
Our families
Simon Gook
Brian Comer at Comer Homes, for the use of Princess Park Manor
Neal Saint at Saints Photographic
Bullies Ballerinas Sarah Newton and Pearl Jordan
Angie Roberts
London Central YMCA Robin Gargrave and Judy Difiore
Professor Craig Sharp
Dr Mark Stillwell
Sylvia Baddeley
Monica McKnight
The Centre for Nutritional Medicine – Dr Beverley Carey, Dr Adam Carey, Dian Mills
Dr Yehudi Gordon
Diane Casewell
Ilkay Arslan and Christine Cremer

EQUIPMENT SUPPLIERS
Reebok
Moda Prima clothing from Pentland Sports, Nashville, USA
Ultratone
Arasys, and The Beauty Suite, W1
Bolton Stirland
WaterRower
Pegasus Pushchairs
Elizabeth Mortlock at Not Only for Maternity
Blooming Marvellous
Gap Kids
Ultimate Fitness, London
Homebase

AND:
Evelyn Pascal at Harland Publishing
Robin Ford at Cell Structures
Anthea Lee at New Nation
Clarins, Jan Marini, Elizabeth Arden, Gatineau, Thalgo, Roc, Higher Nature,
Universal Contour Wrap
Kay Hunter
Rita Owen
Jack Buxton